# Medical Genetics at a Glance

# Medical Genetics at a Glance

## DORIAN J. PRITCHARD

BSc, Dip Gen, PhD, CBiol, MIBiol
Lecturer in Human Genetics (retired)
University of Newcastle-upon-Tyne
UK
Visiting Lecturer in Medical Genetics
International Medical University
Kuala Lumpur
Malaysia

## BRUCE R. KORF

MD, PhD
Wayne H. and Sara Crewes Finley Professor of Genetics
Chairman of Department of Genetics
University of Alabama
Birmingham
Alabama
USA

**Blackwell**
Science

© 2003 by Blackwell Science Ltd
a Blackwell Publishing Company
Editorial Offices:
Osney Mead, Oxford OX2 0EL, UK
    Tel: +44 (0)1865 206206
Blackwell Science, Inc., 350 Main Street, Malden, MA 02148-5018, USA
    Tel: +1 781 388 8250
Blackwell Science Asia Pty, 54 University Street, Carlton, Victoria 3053, Australia
    Tel: +61 (0)3 9347 0300
Blackwell Wissenschafts Verlag, Kurfürstendamm 57, 10707 Berlin, Germany
    Tel: +49 (0)30 32 79 060

First published 2003

Library of Congress Cataloging-in-Publication Data

  Pritchard, D. J. (Dorian J.)
    Medical genetics at a glance / Dorian Pritchard, Bruce R. Korf.
       p. ; cm.
  Includes bibliographical references and index.
    ISBN 0-632-06372-6
  1. Medical genetics.   2. Genetics.   3. Developmental biology.
    [DNLM: 1. Genetics, Medical.   2. Genetics.   QZ 50 P961m   2002]
  I. Korf, Bruce R.   II. Title.
    RB155 .P6965   2002
    616′.042—dc21

2002009523

ISBN 0-632-06372-6

A catalogue record for this title is available from the British Library

Set in 9/11.5 pt Times by SNP Best-set Typesetter Ltd, Hong Kong
Printed and bound in the United Kingdom by Ashford Colour Press, Gosport

For further information on Blackwell Publishing, visit our website:
www.blackwellpublishing.com

# Contents

# Preface

This book is written primarily for medical students seeking a summary of genetics and its medical applications, but it should be of value also to advanced students in the biosciences, paramedical scientists, established medical doctors and health professionals who need to extend or update their knowledge. It should be of especial value to those preparing for examinations.

Medical genetics is unusual in that, whereas its fundamentals usually form part of first-year medical teaching within basic biology, those aspects that relate to inheritance may be presented as an aspect of reproductive biology. Clinical issues usually form a part of later instruction, extending into the postgraduate years. This book is therefore presented in three parts, which can be taken together as a single course, or separately as components of several courses. Chapters are, however, intended to be read in essentially the order of presentation, as concepts and specialized vocabulary are developed progressively.

There are many excellent introductory textbooks in our subject, but none, so far as we know, is at the same time so comprehensive and so succinct. We believe the relative depth of treatment of topics appropriately reflects the importance of these matters in current thinking.

Dorian Pritchard
Bruce Korf

# Acknowledgements

We thank thousands of students, for the motivation they provided by their enthusiastic reception of the lectures on which these chapters are based. We appreciate also the interest and support of many colleagues, but special mention should be made of the constructive criticisms of Paul Brennan. DP wishes to pay tribute to the memory of Ian Cross for his friendship and professional support over many years and for his advice on the chapters dealing with cytogenetics. We thank the staff of Blackwell Publishing for their encouragement and tactful guidance throughout the production of this book.

## Figure acknowledgements

**8 Protein synthesis**
Figure 8: Pritchard DJ (1986) *Foundations of Developmental Genetics*, p.157. Taylor & Francis, London.

**13 The place of genetics in medicine**
Figure 13 (Expression of the major categories of genetic disease in relation to development): Gelehrter TD, Collins FS & Ginsburg D (1998) *Principles of Medical Genetics*, 2nd edn, p.4. Lippincott, Williams and Wilkins, Philadelphia.

**22 Multifactorial threshold traits**
Figure 22 (The threshold model applied to creation of cleft palate): Fraser FC (1977) Relation of animal studies to the problem in man. In: Wilson JG & Clarke-Fraser F (eds) *Handbook of Teratology*, vol. 1, pp. 75–96. Plenum Press, New York.

**26 Allele frequency**
Figure 26: Bodmer WF & Cavalli-Sforza LL (1976) *Genetics, Evolution and Man*. WH Freeman, New York.

# 1 Basic biology

## Control points for gene expression within the cell

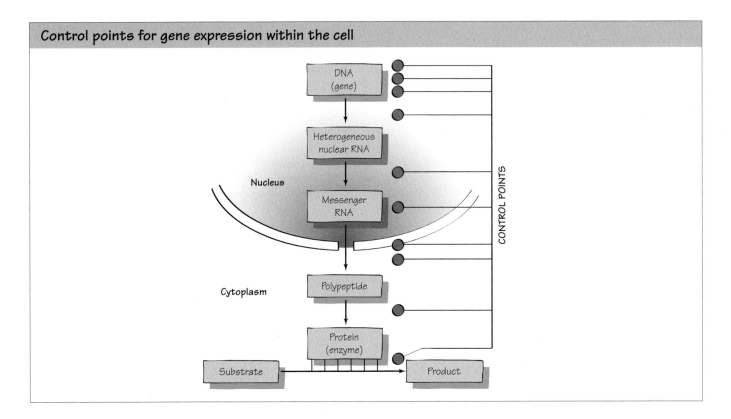

## The case for genetics

Medicine is currently in a state of transformation, created by the convergence of two major aspects of technological advance. The first is the explosion in information technology and the second, the rapidly expanding science of genetics. The likely outcome is that within the foreseeable future we will see the introduction of a new kind of medicine, **individualized medicine**, tailored uniquely to the personal needs of each patient.

Clinicians currently use family histories and genetic testing to identify patients for further evaluation and for guidance on their management. Recognition of the precise (molecular) nature of a disorder enables correct interpretation of ambiguous symptoms. Some diseases, such as hypertension (high blood pressure), have many causes, for which a variety of treatments may be possible. Identification of precise cause would allow clinicians to give personal guidance on the avoidance of adverse stimuli and enable precise targeting of the disease with personally appropriate medications. At the time of writing (2002) more than 5000 people worldwide have received '**gene therapy**', in which attempts have been made to correct errors associated with inherited deficiencies by introduction of normal genes into their cells.

**Pharmacogenetics** is the study of differential responses to unusual biochemicals. For genetic reasons, some individuals are hypersensitive to standard doses of commonly prescribed drugs, while others respond poorly. Genetic insight will guide physicians in the correct prescription of doses while discoveries in other areas of genetics are stimulating development of new kinds of medication. The field of **pharmacoge-**

nomics involves the genetic engineering of pharmaceuticals. Human genes, such as those for insulin and interferon are introduced into microorganisms, field crops and farm animals and these species used as living factories for production of the human proteins. Genomics is also leading to the elucidation of molecular pathways of disease and the ability to design drugs to target specific steps in these pathways.

In research into human diseases, **disease analogues** can be created in laboratory animals by targeted deletion of genes of interest. This approach has been used to create animal models for a wide variety of diseases such as cystic fibrosis and neurofibromatosis.

Some of these topics are outside the scope of this book, but the reader should have no doubt that the medicine of the future, the medicine he or she will practice, will rely very heavily on the insights provided by genetics.

## Overview of Part I

Although genetics is essentially about the transmission of harmful versions of genes from one generation to the next, it encompasses a great deal more. Part I covers the basic biology necessary for its understanding.

### The cell (Chapter 2)

Typically every cell in our bodies contains a pair of each of our genes and these are controlled and expressed in molecular terms *at the level of the cell*. During embryonic development cells in different parts of the body become exposed to different influences and acquire divergent properties, as they begin to express different combinations of the 30–40 000 gene pairs they each contain. Nevertheless, most cells have a similar basic structure and composition, as described in Chapter 2.

## Genetic material (Chapters 3–5)

Most of the biochemical processes of our bodies are catalysed by enzymes and their amino acid sequences are defined by the genes. Genes are coded messages written into an enormously long molecule called **DNA**. This is elaborately coiled and in growing tissue is found alternately extended or tightly contracted.

The DNA is distributed between 23 pairs of homologous **chromosomes**. In a normal woman two of these are large **X-chromosomes**. A normal man also has 46 chromosomes, but in place of one X is a much smaller **Y**, that carries the single gene responsible for triggering male development.

## Gene expression (Chapters 6–8)

The means by which the information contained in the DNA is interpreted is so central to our understanding, that the phrase: *'DNA makes RNA makes protein'*; or, more correctly: **'DNA makes heterogeneous nuclear RNA, which makes messenger RNA, which makes polypeptide, which makes protein';** has become accepted as the **'central dogma'** of molecular biology. The production of the protein product of any gene can potentially be controlled at many steps (see figure).

## Cell division and formation of eggs and sperm
(Chapters 9 and 10)

Body growth involves individual cells replicating their components, dividing in half, expanding and doing the same again. This sequence is called **the cell cycle** and it involves two critical events: **replication** of chromosomal DNA, and segregation of the duplicated chromosomes by **mitosis**.

A modified version of mitosis results in cells with only one, instead of two, sets of chromosomes. This is **meiosis**, which plays a critical part in the creation of the gametes.

## Embryonic development (Chapters 11 and 12)

Fertilization of an egg by a sperm restores the normal chromosome number in the resultant **zygote**. This proliferates to become a hollow ball that **implants** in the maternal uterus. Development proceeds until birth, normally at around 38 weeks, but all the body organs are present in miniature by 6–8 weeks. Thereafter embryogenesis mainly involves **growth** and **differentiation** of cell types. At **puberty** development of the organs of reproduction is restimulated and the individual attains physical maturity.

## Genotype and phenotype

**Genotype** is the word geneticists use for the genetic endowment a person has inherited. **Phenotype** is our word for the anatomical, physiological and psychological complex we recognize as an individual.

People have diverse phenotypes partly because they inherited different genotypes, but an equally important factor is what we can loosely describe as 'environment'. This includes nutrients derived from the bodies of our mothers, growing space, our postnatal feeding and experience, sunlight, exercise, etc. A valuable concept is summarized in the statement: *'Phenotype is the product of interaction between genotype, environment and time'*; or:

Phenotype = Genotype × Environment × Time

**Practically every aspect of phenotype has both genetic and environmental components.** This is a point well worth remembering when we consider the possible causes of any disease, and an issue we address more closely in Part II.

## 2 The cell

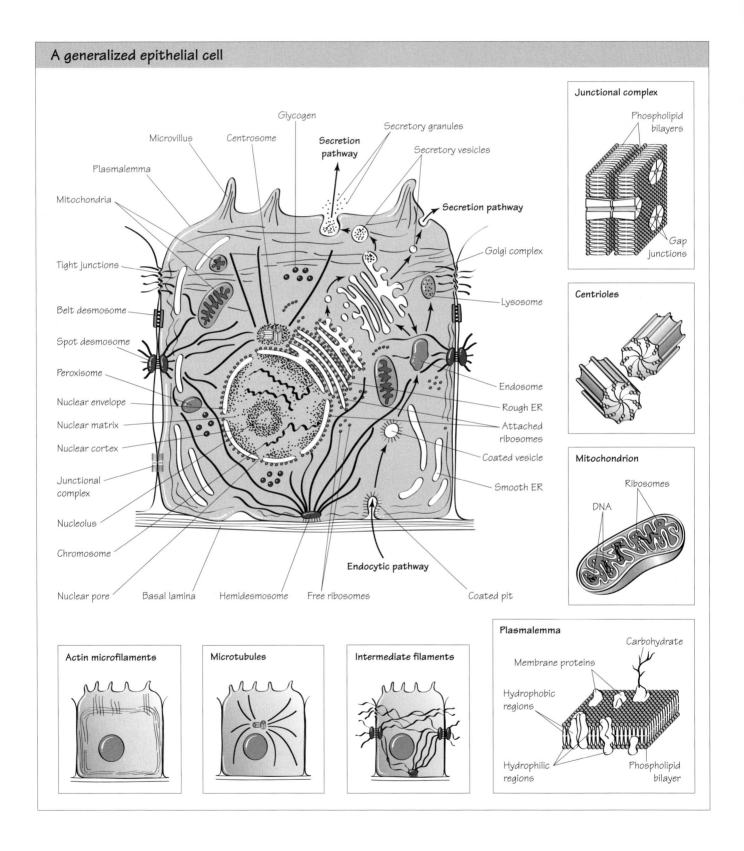

**A generalized epithelial cell**

Glycogen

Microvillus    Centrosome

Plasmalemma

Mitochondria

Tight junctions

Belt desmosome

Spot desmosome

Peroxisome

Nuclear envelope

Nuclear matrix

Nuclear cortex

Junctional
complex

Nucleolus

Chromosome

Nuclear pore    Basal lamina    Hemidesmosome    Free ribosomes

Secretory granules

**Secretion
pathway**

Secretory vesicles

**Secretion pathway**

Golgi complex

Lysosome

Endosome

Rough ER

Attached
ribosomes

Coated vesicle

Smooth ER

**Endocytic pathway**

Coated pit

**Junctional complex**

Phospholipid
bilayers

Gap
junctions

**Centrioles**

**Mitochondrion**

Ribosomes

DNA

**Actin microfilaments**

**Microtubules**

**Intermediate filaments**

**Plasmalemma**

Carbohydrate

Membrane proteins

Hydrophobic
regions

Hydrophilic
regions

Phospholipid
bilayer

## Overview

The cell is the basic functional component of the body. Its **nucleus** is both the repository of the vast majority of the genetic information of that individual and the centre of activity involving its expression. There are many different types of cell (e.g. epithelial, liver, nerve, etc.) and the several kinds of **organelles** and multitudes of soluble enzymes contained within their **cytoplasms** carry out the numerous differentiated aspects of metabolism characteristic of each cell type.

## The plasma membrane

The **plasma membrane**, or **plasmalemma**, is a barrier to water-soluble molecules and defines the interface between the interior and exterior of the cell. It is basically a double, side-by-side array of phospholipid molecules forming a sheet of hydrophobic lipid sandwiched between two sheets of hydrophilic phosphate groups. Within the plasmalemma are a variety of proteins positioned with their hydrophobic regions within the lipid interior and their hydrophilic regions at either surface. **Microvilli** (singular: **microvillus**) are extensions of the apical plasmalemma that provide an increased surface for molecular exchange.

## The nucleus

The genetic information is carried on the **chromosomes** (see Chapter 3) suspended in the **nuclear matrix**. This is a mesh of proteinaceous material densest close to the nuclear envelope where it is called the **nuclear cortex**.

The **nucleolus** is a morphologically distinct region within the nucleus specialized for production of **ribonucleic acid** components of the **ribosomes (rRNA)**. A typical human nucleus contains a single large nucleolus, which at interphase (see Chapter 9) contains the **nucleolar organizer regions** of the acrocentric chromosomes (see Chapters 3 and 38).

The nucleus is bounded by a double membrane called the **nuclear envelope**, perforated by **nuclear pores**.

## The cytoplasm

The **cytoplasm** consists of a gel-like material called the **cytosol**. This contains deposits of glycogen, lipid droplets and free ribosomes (see Chapter 8) and is permeated by an array of interconnected filaments and tubules that form the **cytoskeleton**. The latter has three major structural elements: **microtubules**, **microfilaments** and **intermediate filaments**.

**Microtubules** are straight tubes built from alternating molecules of α- and β-**tubulin**. They radiate from a structure called the **centrosome,** which contains a pair of cylindrical structures called **centrioles** with a characteristic nine-unit structure. (Similar structures occur as **basal bodies** of cilia.) The microtubular network is important in the maintenance of cell shape, separation of the chromosomes during cell division and movement of cilia and sperm.

**Microfilaments** are double-stranded polymers of the protein **actin** distributed mainly near the cell periphery and involved in cell movement and change of cell shape.

**Intermediate filaments** are tubular structures that link the desmosomes. They are composed of one of five or more different proteins, depending on cell type.

**Mitochondria** (singular: **mitochondrion**) are the largest and most abundant of the cytoplasmic organelles. Their main function is the production of energy through synthesis of ATP. They are semiautonomous and self-replicating, each containing ribosomes and up to 10 or more copies of a circular strand of **mitochondrial DNA** carrying the mitochondrial genes (see Chapter 20). They contain the enzymes of the tricarboxylic acid (TCA) cycle and a major fraction of those involved in the oxidation of fatty acids.

**Peroxisomes** are partially responsible for detoxification of foreign compounds such as ethanol, but their major role is the oxidation of fatty acids.

## The secretion pathway

The **endoplasmic reticulum** (**ER**) is a major site of protein and lipid synthesis and represents the beginning of the secretion pathway for proteins. It is a bulky maze of membrane-bound channels continuous with the nuclear envelope. Close to the nucleus it holds bound ribosomes and is known as '**rough ER**'. Away from the nucleus it lacks ribosomes and is called '**smooth ER**'. The ER also plays a role in neutralizing toxins.

Proteins synthesized in the ER are passed to the **Golgi complex** for further processing. This is a series of stacked, flattened vesicles. They are then collected in **storage vesicles** or **secretory vesicles** for **exocytosis**, i.e. release from the cell, in response to external stimuli.

## Endocytosis

**Endocytosis** is the internalization and subsequent processing of constituents of the surrounding medium. Small particles are taken into vesicles by **receptor-mediated pinocytosis,** which involves internalization of surface bound material through formation of a **coated pit**. Larger particles are bound to membrane receptors and engulfed as **phagocytic vacuoles**; solutes are taken in by **fluid-phase pinocytosis**. The content of both pinocytic and phagocytic vesicles is usually delivered to the **lysosomes** for breakdown by enzymes called **lysozymes**. During this transfer the vesicles are sometimes referred to as **endosomes**.

## Cell junctions

**Tight junctions** create a seal between the apical environment of epithelial cells and their basolateral surfaces. **Belt desmosomes** are elongated layers of fibres that assist in the binding together of adjacent cells, together with **spot desmosomes**, which are localized points of adhesion. **Hemidesmosomes** link epithelial cells to their basal lamina, which is a specialized derivative of the **extracellular matrix**. **Gap junctions** are grouped in **junctional complexes**. Each of these contains a pore-permitting molecular communication between adjacent cells.

## Medical issues

Several inherited diseases result from deficiencies in specific lysozymes, including Tay–Sachs, Fabry and Gaucher diseases. Familial hypercholesterolaemia can result from failure of internalization of lipoprotein. Peroxisomes are absent in Zellweger syndrome. Disorders of the mitochondria are described in Chapter 20.

Many therapeutic drugs act on receptors located in the plasma membrane. Microtubule assembly is disrupted by the anticancer agents, *vincristine* and *vinblastine*, as well as *colchicine,* which is used to arrest cells at metaphase of mitosis (see Chapter 9) for examination of the chromosomes (see Chapters 3, 14, 15, 28 and 38). *Clofibrate*, used clinically to lower serum lipoprotein levels, acts by inducing formation of extra peroxisomes.

# 3 The chromosomes

## The basis of chromosome structure

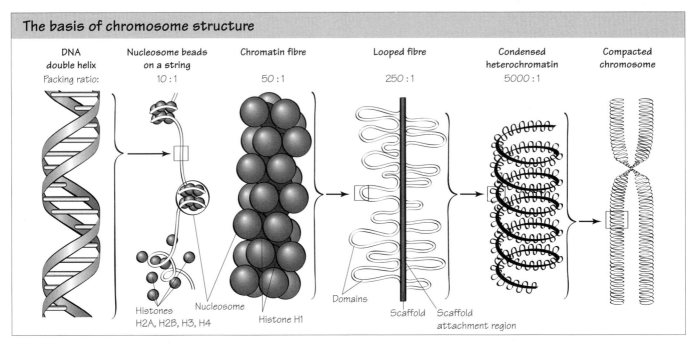

DNA double helix — Packing ratio:

| DNA double helix | Nucleosome beads on a string 10:1 | Chromatin fibre 50:1 | Looped fibre 250:1 | Condensed heterochromatin 5000:1 | Compacted chromosome |

Histones H2A, H2B, H3, H4 — Nucleosome — Histone H1 — Domains — Scaffold — Scaffold attachment region

## A typical chromosome at metaphase of mitosis

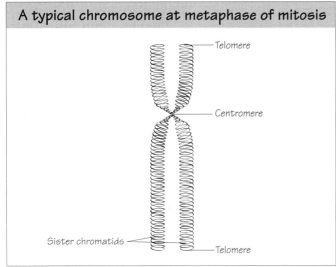

Telomere — Centromere — Sister chromatids — Telomere

## The basis of chromosome banding

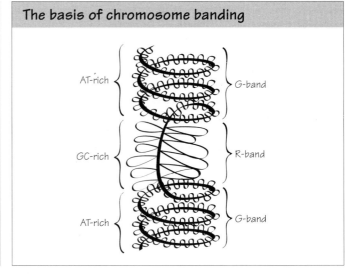

AT-rich — G-band
GC-rich — R-band
AT-rich — G-band

## Overview

The word 'chromosome' means 'coloured body', referring to the capacity of these structures to take up certain histological stains more effectively than other cell structures. Each chromosome is composed of an extremely long molecule of DNA complexed with proteins and RNA to form a substance known as **chromatin**. They disperse throughout the nucleus during **interphase** of the cell cycle (i.e. when the cell is not dividing), but become compacted during **mitosis** and **meiosis** (see Chapters 9 and 10). DNA is packaged as chromosomes probably because packaging facilitates segregation of complete sets of genes into daughter cells at mitosis and packing into sperm heads following meiosis.

The staining properties of the chromosomes are utilized in diagnosis for their general visualization, for their individual identification and for the elucidation of chromosomal abnormalities. We can distinguish lightly staining regions designated **euchromatin**, from densely staining **heterochromatin**. Diagnostic aspects are dealt with in Chapters 14, 15 and 38.

The genetic information, or **genome**, is carried in encoded form in the sequence of bases in the DNA (see Chapters 4–8). The vast majority of this information is in the nucleus, on chromosomes, but a small portion is in the form of naked loops of DNA within each mitochondrion in the cytoplasm. Nuclei are present in practically every cell of the body, the exceptions including red blood cells and the cells of the eye lens.

A typical human nucleus contains around 2 m of DNA divided between 23 pairs of chromosomes, giving an average of about 4 cm per chromosome. But prior to cell division this is reduced to less than 5 μm (0.005 mm) by intricate coiling and packing.

## Chromatin structure

In each chromosome the DNA strand is wound twice around globular aggregates of eight histone proteins to form **nucleosomes**, the whole appearing as a **beaded string structure**. The proteins composing the **nucleosome core particle** are *two* molecules each of histones **H2A**, **H2B**, **H3** and **H4**. Histones are positively charged and so can make ionic bonds with negatively charged phosphate groups in the DNA. The amino acid sequences of histones show close to 100% identity across species, indicating their great importance in maintenance of chromatin structure and function. Each nucleosome accommodates about 200 base pairs of DNA and effectively reduces the length of the DNA strand to one tenth.

The beaded string is then further coiled into a **solenoid**, or spiral coil, with five to six nucleosomes per turn, the structure being maintained by mediation of *one* molecule of histone **H1** per nucleosome. Formation of the solenoid decreases the effective length of the DNA strand by another factor of five, yielding an overall 'packing ratio' of about 50. This is the probable state of euchromatin at interphase in regions where the genes are not being expressed.

During mitosis and meiosis the chromosomes are condensed, a further 100-fold, achieving packing ratios of around 5000. The chromatin fibre is thought to be folded into a series of loops radiating from a central **scaffold** of **non-histone chromosomal (NHC) proteins** that bind to specific base sequences scattered along the DNA strand. Compaction of the chromosome probably involves contraction of these NHC proteins.

One of the most important of the scaffold proteins is **topoisomerase II**, a DNA-nicking-closing enzyme that permits the uncoiling of the two strands of the DNA double helix necessary for the relaxation of DNA supercoils during replication or transcription (see Chapters 5 and 7). Topoisomerase II binds to **scaffold attachment regions** that are AT-rich (i.e. contain more than 65% of the bases A and T; see Chapter 4). It is believed that each loop may possibly act as an independent functional domain with respect to DNA replication or transcription.

The looped fibre is then further coiled to create the fully condensed heterochromatin of a chromosome at cell division.

## Chromosome banding

Some parts of the compacted chromosome stain densely with Giemsa stain to create **G-bands**. These contain tightly packed, small loops because the scaffold attachment regions there are close together. They replicate late in S-phase (see Chapter 9) and are relatively inactive in transcription. Bands that stain lightly with Giemsa stain, **R-bands**, contain more loosely packed loops, are relatively rich in bases G and C and show most transcriptional activity. Differences between banding patterns of chromosomes allow their identification (see Chapter 38).

## The centromere

When visible in early mitosis each chromosome is composed of two identical structures called **sister chromatids** connected at a **primary constriction**. This consists of a non-duplicated stretch of DNA called the **centromere** that duplicates during early anaphase of mitosis (see Chapter 9).

An organelle called the **kinetochore** becomes located on each side of each centromere in early prophase of mitosis and facilitates polymerization of **tubulin** dimers to form the **microtubules** of the **mitotic spindle**.

## The telomeres

The term '**telomere**' refers to the specialized end of a chromosome. Specific telomeric proteins bind to this structure to provide a cap (see Chapter 5).

The telomeres have several probable functions: preventing the abnormal end-to-end fusion of chromosomes, ensuring complete replication of chromosome extremities, assisting with chromosome pairing in **meiosis** (see Chapter 10) and helping to establish the internal structure of the nucleus during interphase by linking the chromosomes to the nuclear membrane.

## Euchromatin and heterochromatin

Euchromatin is compacted during cell division, but relaxes into an open conformation during interphase. In compacted chromosomes it constitutes the palely staining R-bands and contains the majority of the structural genes.

Heterochromatin is densely compacted at cell division and remains compacted at interphase. It is largely concentrated around the nuclear periphery and nucleolus and is relatively inactive in transcription. **Constitutive heterochromatin** is common to all cells of the body, while **facultative heterochromatin** varies, representing regions of the genome that are expressed differentially in the different cell types.

# 4 DNA structure

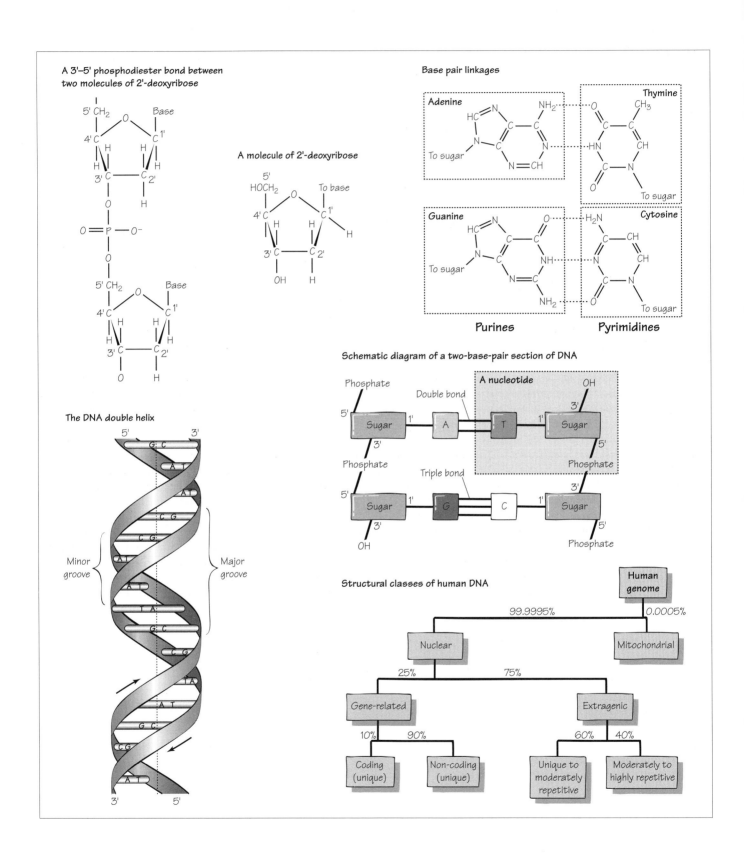

A 3'–5' phosphodiester bond between two molecules of 2'-deoxyribose

A molecule of 2'-deoxyribose

Base pair linkages

Adenine        Thymine
Guanine        Cytosine

Purines        Pyrimidines

The DNA double helix

Minor groove        Major groove

Schematic diagram of a two-base-pair section of DNA

Phosphate
Double bond        A nucleotide        OH
Phosphate        Triple bond
OH        Phosphate

Structural classes of human DNA

Human genome

99.9995%        0.0005%

Nuclear        Mitochondrial

25%        75%

Gene-related        Extragenic

10%        90%        60%        40%

Coding (unique)        Non-coding (unique)        Unique to moderately repetitive        Moderately to highly repetitive

## Overview

As we learnt in Chapter 3, the chromosomes are composed essentially of **DNA**, which contains coded instructions for synthesis of every protein in the body. DNA consists of millions of nucleotides within two interlinked, coiled chains. Each nucleotide contains one of four bases and it is the sequence of these bases that contains the coded instructions.

Each base on one chain is matched by a complementary partner on the other, and each sequence provides a template for synthesis of a copy of the other. Synthesis of new DNA is called **replication** (see Chapter 5).

The unit of length of DNA is the **base pair** (**bp**) with 1000 bp in a **kilobase** (**kb**) and 1000,000 bp in a **megabase** (**Mb**). A typical human body cell contains nearly 7000 Mb of DNA.

## The structure of DNA

We can imagine the structure of DNA as like an extremely long, flexible ladder that has been twisted right-handed (like a corkscrew) by coiling around a telegraph pole. Each 'upright' of the ladder is a series of **deoxyribose** sugar molecules linked together by phosphate groups attached to their 3′ ('three prime') and 5′ ('five prime') carbon atoms. At the bottom of one upright is a 3′ carbon atom carrying a free hydroxyl (—OH) group and, at the top, a 5′ carbon carrying a free phosphate group. On the other upright this orientation is reversed.

The 'rungs' of the ladder are pairs of nitrogenous **bases** of two types, **purines** and **pyrimidines**. The purines are **adenine** (**A**) and **guanine** (**G**) and the pyrimidines are **cytosine** (**C**) and **thymine** (**T**). The bases are attached to the 1′ carbon of each sugar. Each unit of purine or pyrimidine base together with one attached sugar and one phosphate group constitute a **nucleotide**. A section of double-stranded DNA is therefore essentially two linked, coiled chains of nucleotides. This **double helix** has a **major groove** corresponding to the gap between adjacent sections of the sugar-phosphate chains and a **minor groove** along the row of bases. There are 10 pairs of nucleotides per complete turn of the helix.

The pairs of bases of the 'rungs' are hydrogen-bonded together and since both A and T have two sites available for bonding while C and G each have three. *A always pairs with T on the opposite strand and C with G.* This **base pairing** (known as Watson–Crick base pairing) is very specific and ensures that the strands are normally precisely complementary to one another. Thus if one strand reads 5′-CGAT-3′, the complementary strand must read 3′-GCTA-5′ in the same direction, or 5′-ATCG-3′ if we obey the normal rule of describing the sequence from 5′ to 3′. The number of A residues in a section of DNA is therefore always equal to the number of T residues; similarly, the number of C residues always equals the number of G (Chargaff's rule).

## The centromeres

Centromeric DNA contains short sequences of bases repeated many times 'in tandem array'. The sequences vary between chromosomes, but there are substantial regions of homology. The most important component is a 171-bp repeat called **alpha-satellite DNA**. This is AT-rich and contains a binding site for a protein contained within the kinetochore. The latter is responsible for assembly of the microtubules of the spindle apparatus.

## The telomeres

In contrast to the centromeric repeats, telomeric sequences are the same in all human chromosomes and similar to those in other species. Human telomeric DNA consists of long arrays of tandem repeats of the sequence 5′-GGGTTA-3′ extending for several hundred bases on each chromosome end. Most of this is double stranded, with 3′-CCCAAT-5′ on the complementary strand, but the extreme 3′ end is single stranded and believed to loop around and invade the double helix several kilobases away. The triple-stranded structure so formed is stabilized by binding telomere-specific protein (see Chapter 5).

## Structural classes of human DNA

The human *haploid* genome contains probably 30–40 000 nuclear genes, i.e. coding sequences and their associated control elements, in addition to 37 (including those for mitochondrial tRNA: see Chapter 6) within the mitochondrial genome. However, *the nuclear genome represents no more than 3% of nuclear DNA*, the remainder having no coding function. This includes **introns** that interrupt the coding **exons** of most genes, plus the 75% of human nuclear DNA that is extragenic, i.e. outside or between the genes. Of the latter, 60% is of unique sequence or moderately repetitive, while 40% is moderately to highly repetitive.

The highly repetitive fraction includes **microsatellite** and **minisatellite DNA**, which differ in the length of the repeat. Satellite DNA is so-called because its unusual AT : GC ratio gives it a buoyant density that differs from the bulk of the DNA. This causes it to separate out as a 'satellite band' when mechanically sheared whole DNA is subjected to density gradient centrifugation.

## Medical and legal issues

Microsatellite DNA is scattered throughout the genome and is useful for tracking the inheritance of disease alleles of closely linked genes. Minisatellite DNA is concentrated near the centromeres and telomeres, so is less useful for tracking genes, but, since it is highly variable, it is used for producing **DNA fingerprints**. These play an exceptionally important role in paternity testing and forensic identification (see Chapter 46).

# 5 DNA replication

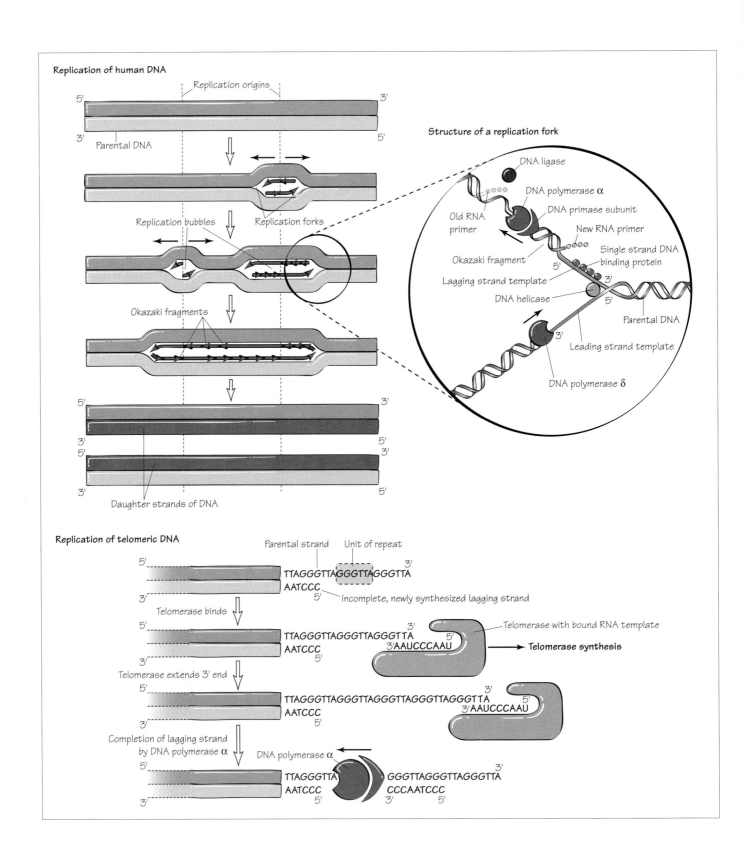

**Replication of human DNA**

Replication origins

5'

3'
Parental DNA

5'

3'

5'

Replication bubbles    Replication forks

Okazaki fragments

5'                              3'
3'                              5'
5'                              3'

3'                              5'
Daughter strands of DNA

**Structure of a replication fork**

DNA ligase
DNA polymerase α
Old RNA primer
DNA primase subunit
New RNA primer
Okazaki fragment
Single strand DNA binding protein
5'
Lagging strand template
3'
DNA helicase
5'
Parental DNA
3'
Leading strand template
DNA polymerase δ

**Replication of telomeric DNA**

Parental strand    Unit of repeat

5'
TTAGGGTTAGGGTTAGGGTTA    3'
AATCCC
3'
5'
Incomplete, newly synthesized lagging strand

Telomerase binds

5'
TTAGGGTTAGGGTTAGGGTTA    3'
AATCCC                    3'AAUCCCAAU
3'                        5'
Telomerase with bound RNA template
Telomerase synthesis

Telomerase extends 3' end

5'
TTAGGGTTAGGGTTAGGGTTAGGGTTAGGGTTA    3'
AATCCC                                5'
3'                        3'AAUCCCAAU
5'

Completion of lagging strand by DNA polymerase α
DNA polymerase α

5'
TTAGGGTTA    GGGTTAGGGTTAGGGTTA    3'
AATCCC       CCCAATCCC
3'
5'    3'    5'

## Overview

Cells multiply by the process of mitosis, but so that genetic information is not lost, the whole of the nuclear genome is first duplicated. This occurs during **S-phase** of the **cell cycle** (see Chapter 9). S-phase lasts about 8 h. The DNA at the centromeres of the chromosomes is replicated in the middle of mitosis, just before chromosome segregation. Mitochondrial DNA is replicated out of phase with nuclear DNA.

Although the overall sequence of events during replication of nuclear DNA in higher organisms (eukaryotes) is similar to that in bacteria (prokaryotes), the details are subtly different. In eukaryotes replication takes place while the (nuclear) DNA remains in nucleosome configuration (see Chapter 3).

## Replication

GC-rich sections of the DNA, recognizable as euchromatic R-bands in condensed chromatin (see Chapter 3), contain 'housekeeping genes' that operate in every cell. These sections replicate in the early S-phase (see Chapter 9). The heterochromatic AT-rich G-bands contain few genes and replicate in late S-phase (see Chapter 3). Genes in AT-rich regions that code for differentiated properties and operate in some cells only are found in facultative heterochromatin (see Chapter 3). This is replicated early in those cells in which the genes are expressed and late in those in which they are not.

The place on the DNA helix which first unwinds to begin replication is called the **replication origin**. Here the double strand is split open by a **helicase** enzyme to expose the base sequences. Replication proceeds along the single strands at about 40–50 nucleotides per second, simultaneously in both directions. In higher organisms there are many replication origins spaced about 50–300 kb apart. The resulting separations of the DNA strand are called **replication bubbles**, at each end of which is a **replication fork**.

New DNA is synthesized by enzymes called **DNA polymerases,** from **deoxyribonucleotide triphosphates** (**ATP**, **GTP**, etc.), which in the process are converted into monophosphate nucleotides (**AMP**, **GMP**, etc.). The release and hydrolysis of pyrophosphate from the triphosphates provides energy for the reaction and ensures it is virtually irreversible, making DNA a relatively very robust molecule.

All DNA polymerases can build new DNA only in the 5′ to 3′ direction, which means they must move along their **template strands** from 3′ to 5′. Replication can therefore occur continuously from the origin of replication along only one strand, called the **leading strand**. The other strand is called the **lagging strand** and, because of the orientation of the sugars along this strand, replication takes place only in short stretches. The new sections of DNA along the lagging strand are typically 100–200 bases long and are known as **Okazaki fragments**. Following their synthesis they are linked together by action of the enzyme **DNA ligase**. While awaiting replication the parental single-strand sequence of the lagging strand is temporarily protected by **single-strand binding protein** (or **helix-destabilizing protein**).

Leading strand synthesis requires **DNA polymerase δ**; lagging strand synthesis uses a different enzyme, **DNA polymerase α**. The latter contains a **DNA primase** subunit that produces a short stretch of RNA (see Chapter 6), which acts as a primer for DNA synthesis. Replication of mitochondrial DNA occurs independently of that in the nucleus and utilizes a different set of enzymes, including the mitochondria-specific **DNA polymerase γ**.

The genome contains multiple copies of the five histone genes, from which copious quantities of histones are produced, especially during S-phase. These bind immediately onto the newly replicated DNA.

Since each daughter DNA duplex contains one old strand from the parent molecule and one newly synthesized strand, the replication process is described as **semiconservative**.

## Replication of the telomeres

Synthesis of DNA at the end of the lagging strand is problematical as DNA polymerase α needs to attach beyond the end of the sequence that is being replicated and work proximally, in the 5′-3′ direction. A specialized DNA synthetic enzyme called **telomerase** provides an extension of the lagging strand that enables this to happen.

Telomerase is a ribonucleoprotein that contains an RNA template with the sequence 3′-AAUCCCAAU-3′. This is complementary to one-and-a-half copies of the six-base telomeric DNA repeat, 5′-GGGTTA-3′ (see Chapter 4). The 3′-AAU of the RNA sequence of the telomerase binds to the terminal –TTA-5′ of the template lagging strand, leaving the rest of the RNA sequence exposed. Deoxyribonucleotides then assemble on this RNA template, extending the DNA repeat sequence by one unit. The telomerase then detaches and moves along to the new DNA terminal -TTA-3′, where the process is repeated. When a sufficiently long-terminal repeat has been formed, DNA polymerase α attaches to the single-strand extension and assembles the complementary DNA strand in a proximal 5′-3′ direction back to the old end of the double strand, to which it becomes linked by the action of DNA ligase.

## Repair systems

Occasionally a wrong base is inserted into a growing strand but, fortunately, healthy cells contain **postreplication repair enzymes** and **base mismatch proofreading systems** that correct such errors. These remove and replace the erroneously inserted bases, using the template strand as a guide. These repair systems utilize two additional DNA polymerases: β and ε (see Chapter 29).

## Medical issues

Several cancer-predisposing conditions arise from defects in different aspects of the postreplication repair and mismatch repair systems. These include the chromosome breakage syndrome called **Bloom syndrome**, familial predisposition to breast cancer caused by mutations in the genes **BRCA1** and **BRCA2** and an autosomal dominant form of bowel cancer called **hereditary non-polyposis colon cancer (HNPCC)** (see Chapter 32).

One theory holds that telomeres are reduced in length at every round of mitosis and that the number of repeats they contain may play a role in limiting the number of times a cell can divide. On this theory, abnormally efficient, mutant telomerases may promote the indefinite growth of cancer cells by delaying telomere decay.

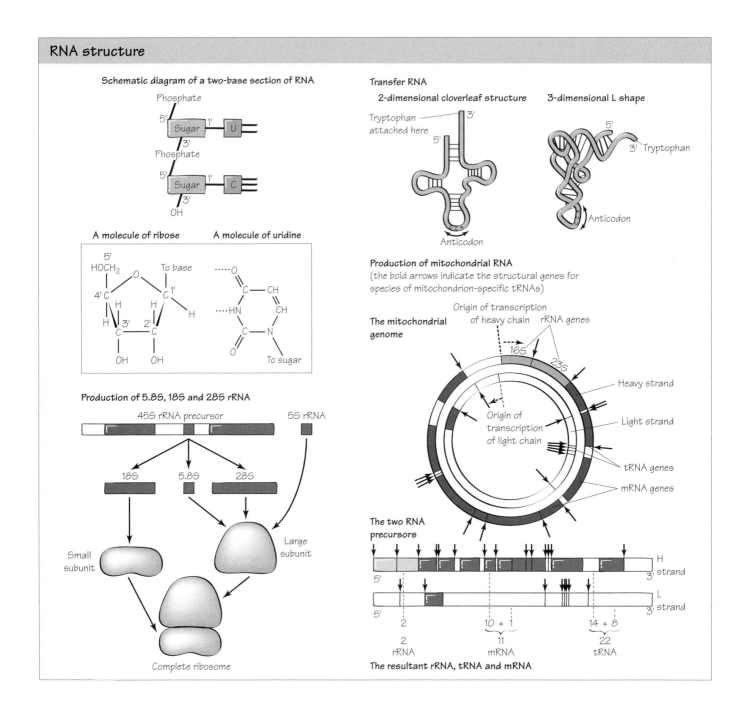

## RNA structure

**Schematic diagram of a two-base section of RNA**

**A molecule of ribose**

**A molecule of uridine**

**Production of 5.8S, 18S and 28S rRNA**

**Transfer RNA**

**2-dimensional cloverleaf structure**

Tryptophan attached here

Anticodon

**3-dimensional L shape**

Tryptophan

Anticodon

**Production of mitochondrial RNA** (the bold arrows indicate the structural genes for species of mitochondrion-specific tRNAs)

The mitochondrial genome

Origin of transcription of heavy chain

rRNA genes

16S

23S

Origin of transcription of light chain

Heavy strand

Light strand

tRNA genes

mRNA genes

The two RNA precursors

H strand

L strand

| 2 | 10 + 1 | 14 + 8 |
| 2 rRNA | 11 mRNA | 22 tRNA |

The resultant rRNA, tRNA and mRNA

## Overview

In Chapter 4 we learnt that DNA is the double-stranded nucleic acid that carries the genetic information we received from our parents and which we pass on to our children. **RNA** is a similar molecule that facilitates the expression of this genetic information within our own cells. The main differences between RNA and DNA are that RNA is (usually) single stranded, **ribose** replaces deoxyribose and **uracil** (U) replaces thymine. In **eukaryotes** (literally organisms with a 'true nucleus', i.e. higher organisms) RNA occurs as six types of molecule: **messenger RNA (mRNA)**, its precursor **heterogeneous nuclear RNA (hnRNA)**, **transfer RNA (tRNA)**, **ribosomal RNA (rRNA)**, **small nuclear RNA (snRNA)** and **mitochondrial RNA (mtRNA)**. Heterogeneous nuclear RNA is characteristic of eukaryotes and is not found in **prokaryotes** (literally 'before the nucleus', e.g. bacteria and viruses). Some viruses use RNA in place of DNA for storage and transfer of genetic information.

## Heterogeneous nuclear and messenger RNA

Heterogeneous nuclear RNA and its derivative mRNA carry genetic information from the nuclear DNA into the cytoplasm.

There are as many species of hnRNA as there are genes, because hnRNA is the direct transcript of the coding sequences of the genome. They are transcribed from the DNA by the enzyme **RNA polymerase II (Pol II)**. Messenger RNA results from the processing of hnRNA, which includes the removal of non-coding **introns** and linking together of the coding **exons** (see Chapter 7). mRNA therefore carries only the coding information of the corresponding species of each hnRNA, plus the flanking leader and trailer, and so is considerably shorter.

## Transfer RNA

Each molecule of transfer RNA consists of about 75 nucleotides linked together in a long chain which, due to internal base pairing, adopts a 'clover leaf' structure, which then twists into an L shape. Transfer RNA is unusual in containing a variety of rarer bases in addition to C, G, A and U, and some of these are modified by methylation. The important feature of tRNA is that each 'charged' molecule carries an amino acid at its 3′ end, while on the middle 'leaf' of the cloverleaf structure are three characteristic bases known as the **anticodon**. The sequence of bases in the anticodon is specifically related to the species of amino acid attached to the 3′ terminus. For example, tRNA with the anticodon 5′-CCA-3′ carries the amino acid tryptophan and no other. It is this specific relationship that forms the basis of translation of the genetic message carried by mRNA (see Chapter 8).

Transfer RNA molecules are transcribed from their coding sequences in DNA by the enzyme **RNA polymerase III (Pol III)**. There are over 40 different tRNA subfamilies, each with several members.

## Ribosomal RNA

Ribosomal RNA consists of several species usually referred to by their sedimentation coefficients in Svedberg units (S), deduced by their speed of centrifugation in a dense aqueous medium.

Each **ribosome** consists of one large and one small subunit. These contain many proteins derived by translation of mRNA, plus RNA that remains untranslated. The term 'ribosomal RNA' refers to the non-translated material. The small ribosomal subunit contains **18S rRNA** and the large subunit **5S, 5.8S** and **28S rRNA**.

Ribosomal RNA is transcribed from DNA by two additional RNA polymerases. **Polymerase I (Pol I)** transcribes 5.8 S, 18 S and 28 S, as one long **45S** transcript which is then cleaved into three sections, so ensuring they are produced in equal quantities. We each carry about 250 copies of the DNA sequence coding for the 45S transcript per haploid genome. These are in five clusters of tandem repeats on the short arms of chromosomes 13, 14, 15, 21 and 22. These are known as the **nucleolar organizer regions**, as their transcription and the subsequent processing of the 45S transcript occurs while they are held within the nucleolus.

There are about 2000 copies of the 5S rRNA gene in at least three clusters on Chromosome 1. These are transcribed by **Pol III** outside the nucleolus and imported for ribosome assembly, along with ribosomal proteins.

## Small nuclear RNA

The conversion of hnRNA into mRNA by the removal of introns occurs in the nucleus in RNA-protein complexes called **spliceosomes**. Each spliceosome has a core of three **small nuclear ribonucleo-proteins** or **snRNPs** (pronounced 'snurps'). Each snRNP contains at least one snRNA and several proteins. There are several hundred different snRNAs, transcribed mainly by Pol II, which are believed to be capable of recognizing specific ribonucleic acid sequences by RNA–RNA base pairing. The most important in hnRNA processing are U1, U2, U4/U6 and U5.

## Mitochondrial RNA

Mitochondrial DNA is in the form of a continuous loop coding for 13 polypeptides, 22 tRNAs and two rRNAs (one 16S, the other 23S). Most genes are on one strand, the **heavy strand**, but a few are on its complement, the **light strand** and *both strands are transcribed*, as two continuous transcripts, by a **mitochondrion-specific RNA polymerase**. This enzyme is coded by a nuclear gene. The long RNA molecules are then cleaved to produce 37 separate RNA species and the mitochondrial, ribosomal and transfer RNAs join forces to translate the 13 mRNAs. Many additional proteins are imported into the mitochondria from the cytoplasm, having been transcribed from nuclear genes.

## Medical issues

Patients with **systemic lupus erythematosus** have antibodies directed against their own snRNP proteins.

## Key sequences in mRNA production

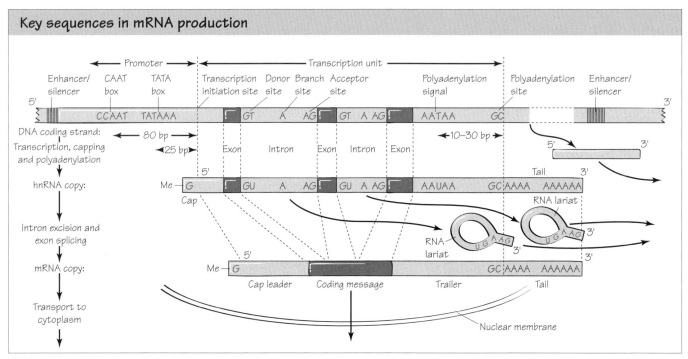

## Transcription by RNA polymerase II

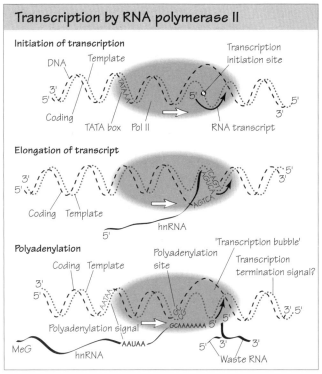

## Intron excision and exon splicing

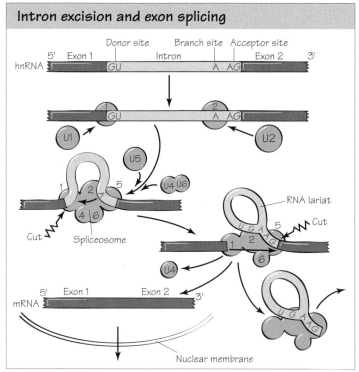

## Overview

Most metabolic processes are catalysed by proteinaceous enzymes. Proteins are also the main structural components of the body and the amino acid sequences of all proteins are coded in the DNA. Conversion of the DNA-encoded information into protein involves transcription into an hnRNA copy, processing into mRNA, translation into polypeptide and elaboration into protein (see Chapter 8).

## The structure of a gene

Eukaryotes differ from prokaryotes in that most of their genes contain redundant DNA that interrupts the coding sequences. These stretches of non-coding DNA are called **introns**, while the coding sequences are called **exons**. In both groups, outside the coding region are a **leader** and **trailer**, plus a variety of transcriptional control sequences.

Genes that code for protein are called 'structural genes' and their transcription is performed by RNA polymerase Pol II. A sequence just 'upstream' (i.e. 5′) of the coding sequence constitutes the **promoter**, which acts as a binding site for **transcription factors** that indicate where Pol II should begin its action.

Among proteins we can distinguish 'housekeeping proteins' present in all cell types and 'luxury proteins' produced for specialized functions. The promoters of genes that code for luxury proteins include a 'TATA box', with a sequence that is a variant of 5′-TATAAA-3′ at about 25 bp upstream of the **transcription initiation site**. Genes that code for 'housekeeping proteins' instead usually have one or more 'GC boxes' in variable positions, containing a variant of 5′-GGGCGG-3′. Another common promoter element is the 'CAAT box' (e.g. 5′-CCAAT-3′) at −80 bp and there are often also **enhancer** and **silencer** sequences some distance away that bind controlling factors, which interact with the promoter by looping of the DNA. Some 'luxury' genes have additional function-specific control elements.

'Downstream' (i.e. 3′) of the transcription initiation site is the **leader sequence**, which is not translated. The coding message follows, usually interrupted by one or more introns and followed by the non-coding **trailer**. At the end of the trailer is the **polyadenylation site** of variable sequence, but defined by 5′-AATAA-3′ (5′-AAUAA-3′ in the RNA transcript), 10–30 bases upstream.

Introns begin with the sequence **GT**A(/G)GAGT and end with a run of Cs or Ts preceding **AG**. The first **GT** (**GU** in the hnRNA) and the last **AG**, together with an **A** residue situated within a relatively standard sequence near the downstream end, are important in intron removal. The 5′ site is known as the **donor** site, the 3′ site is the **acceptor** and the A residue is the **branch** site.

In *prokaryotes* transcription stops at a specific point indicated by an inverted repeat in the trailer, followed by a run of T residues. The adoption of a hairpin loop by base pairing in the mRNA copy brings transcription to an end. An analogous structure exists in histone gene trailers, but *no general transcription termination signal has been identified in eukaryotes*.

## Transcription

Transcription is signalled by assembly of protein transcription factors at the promoter. A molecule of Pol II binds to this complex and splits open the double helix. The complex, now including the enzyme, then moves downstream causing local unwinding and splitting, followed by re-formation of the double helix as it proceeds, creating a 17-bp long **transcription bubble**. When it reaches the transcription initiation point it ejects one transcription factor, acquires another and begins to synthesize RNA.

Using the strand orientated in the 3′-5′ direction (from left to right) as a template, Pol II links ribonucleotides one by one to produce a complementary RNA sequence, orientated with reverse polarity (i.e. 5′ to 3′). In other words, by applying the rules of base pairing to the **template strand** it creates a precise RNA copy of the **coding strand**. The enzyme transcribes through leader, exons, introns and trailer, and (apparently wastefully!) proceeds indefinitely downstream (see above).

## RNA processing

As hnRNA transcripts are synthesized, they are covalently modified to distinguish them as coded messages for later translation into polypeptide. The 5′ end is first capped by addition of 7-methyl GTP in reverse orientation. When the polyadenylation site appears in the hnRNA strand, it is cleaved there and **poly-A polymerase** adds on 100–200 residues of adenylic acid to form the **poly-A tail**. Both the cap and tail probably protect the molecule from degradation, contribute to the 'passport' that allows its export to the cytoplasm and later provide a recognition signal for the ribosome, indicating its availability for translation.

On average, an hnRNA molecule may have about 7000 nucleotides which are reduced to about 1200 in the mRNA by removal of as many as 50 introns. Histone genes are exceptional in having no introns.

The ribonucleoprotein complexes that remove the introns are called **spliceosomes** and they contain several snRNA species (U1–U6), each complexed with specific proteins. U1 snRNP (i.e. ribonucleoprotein containing U1 snRNA) binds to the upstream splice site, guided by a complementary sequence in the U1 snRNA. U2 snRNP binds to the branch site, then becomes linked to the bound U1, causing a loop in the hnRNA. U2 then cuts the hnRNA immediately upstream of **GU** (see above) and joins that upstream cut end of the intron to the junction site, creating a **lariat** shape. The downstream end of the intron is then cut just beyond **AG**, releasing the RNA lariat, and the spliceosome brings together and joins the two exons.

## Medical issues

*Alpha-amanitin* from the death cap mushroom, *Amanita phalloides*, blocks the action of Pol II. Alternative RNA splicing occurs normally in some transcripts, notably in the production of antibodies (see Chapter 33). Many genetic disorders involve errors in RNA splicing. The antibiotic, *rifampicin* (*rifamycin*) blocks bacterial transcription by binding to the prokaryote promoter; *actinomycin* intercalates between G-C pairs.

# 8 Protein synthesis

## The genetic code

Amino acid single
letter code:       A          C          D              E                F                  G
Abbreviation:      Ala        Cys        Asp            Glu              Phe                Gly
Amino acid:        Alanine    Cysteine   Aspartic acid  Glutamic acid    Phenylalanine      Glycine

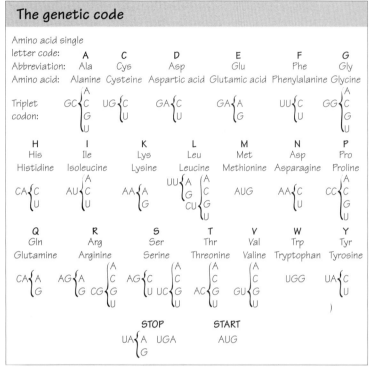

Triplet codon:

| | | | | | |
|---|---|---|---|---|---|
| GC{C G U A | UG{C U | GA{C U | GA{A G | UU{C U | GG{A C G U |

       H          I          K              L                M                  N            P
       His        Ile        Lys            Leu              Met                Asp          Pro
       Histidine  Isoleucine Lysine         Leucine          Methionine         Asparagine   Proline

CA{C U    AU{A C U    AA{A G    UU{A G   CU{A C G U    AUG    AA{C U    CC{A C G U

       Q          R          S              T                V                  W            Y
       Gln        Arg        Ser            Thr              Val                Trp          Tyr
       Glutamine  Arginine   Serine         Threonine        Valine             Tryptophan   Tyrosine

CA{A G    AG{A G   CG{A C G U    AG{C U   UC{A C G U   AC{A C G U   GU{A C G U    UGG    UA{C U

                              STOP                START
                         UA{A G  UGA            AUG

## Setting of the reading frame

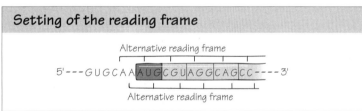

Alternative reading frame

5'---GUGCAA AUG CGU AGG CAG CC----3'

Alternative reading frame

## The peptidyl transferase reaction

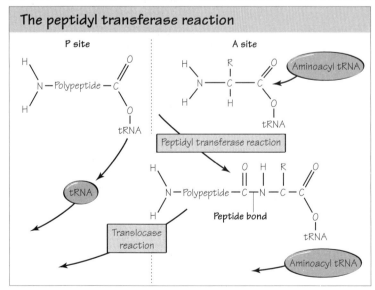

## Translation

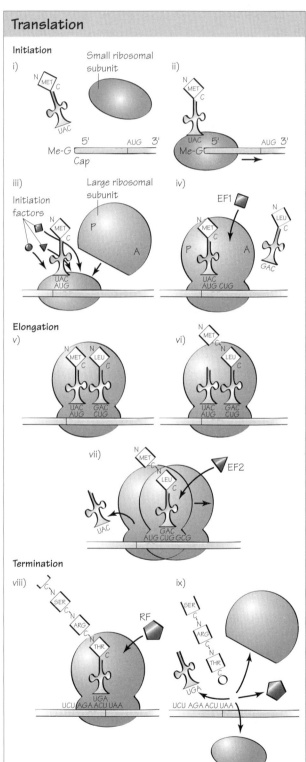

### Initiation

i) Small ribosomal subunit

ii)

iii) Large ribosomal subunit — Initiation factors

iv) EF1

### Elongation

v)

vi)

vii) EF2

### Termination

viii) RF

ix)

## Overview

The main structural components of the body and most of its catalysts are **proteins**, each derived from one or more **polypeptides**. A polypeptide is a chain of amino acids, the sequence of which is determined by that of the bases in the corresponding mRNA, in accordance with '**the genetic code**'. Each amino acid is represented in mRNA by one or more groups of three bases called **triplet codons,** and their interpretation as polypeptide is called **translation**. Messenger RNA is translated from the 5′ to the 3′ end within cytoplasmic **ribosomes**. The resultant polypeptides are then modified into proteins. The functional properties of proteins derive largely from the active groups they display in their tertiary and quaternary conformations.

## The genetic code

Translation requires transfer RNA molecules charged with amino acids appropriate to their anticodon sequences (see Chapter 6). Some amino acids are coded by several codons, only tryptophan and methionine by one each. Three of the 64 possible three-fold combinations of A, C, G and U in the mRNA code for **STOP signals**: **UGA**, **UAG** and **UAA** (see 'The genetic code' in the figure). **AUG** codes for methionine and also acts as a **START signal**, simultaneously determining the amino- (or N-) terminal end of the polypeptide and selecting one of the three possible **reading frames** (see 'Setting of the reading frame' in the figure). The genetic code of mitochondria is slightly different.

## Translation

### Initiation

A small ribosomal subunit containing several **initiation factors** and methionyl tRNA charged with methionine binds to the 5′ cap on the mRNA and then slides along until it finds and engages with the first AUG sequence. The initiation factors are then released, a large ribosomal subunit binds to the small one, and translation begins.

The large ribosomal subunit contains two sites, known as the **A site** (for aminoacyl) and the **P site** (for peptidyl). At the end of initiation the P site contains a charged met-tRNA with its anticodon engaged in the first AUG codon, while the A site is empty.

### Elongation

The appropriate aminoacyl tRNA now becomes located in the A site, as dictated by the adjacent codon in the mRNA, with the help of a soluble **elongation factor** called **EF1**. The **peptidyl transferase reaction** then creates a **peptide bond** between the amino (—NH2) group of the amino acid at the A site and the carboxyl (—COOH) group of that at the P site, while the first tRNA is released.

The **translocase reaction** next promotes expulsion of the uncharged tRNA, moves the ribosome three bases along and translocates the growing peptide from A to P. This requires **elongation factor, EF2**.

Mitochondrial mRNAs are translated by mitochondria-specific tRNAs.

### Termination

Elongation continues until a STOP codon enters the ribosome, all three being recognized by a single multivalent **release factor (RF)**. This modifies the specificity of peptidyl transferase so that a molecule of water is added to the peptide instead. The ribosome is then released and dissociates into its subunits, so freeing the completed polypeptide.

Synthesis of an average polypeptide of 400 amino acids takes about 20 seconds.

As each ribosome vacates the messenger cap another attaches and follows its predecessor, creating a **polyribosome** or **polysome**. The mRNA usually survives for a few hours.

## Protein structure

The amino acid sequence of a polypeptide defines its **primary structure**. The **secondary structure** is the three-dimensional form of parts of the polypeptide: the **α-helix**, the **collagen pro-α helix,** or the **β-pleated sheet**.

**Tertiary structure** is the folded form of the whole polypeptide, composed of different secondary structures.

**Quaternary structure** is the final native conformation of a multimeric protein, e.g. **haemoglobin** is composed of two **α-globin** monomers, **two β-globin** monomers, one molecule of **haem** and an atom of ferrous iron. **Collagen fibres** are cables of many triple helices, each formed as a rope of three pro-α helices.

Structure is frequently maintained by **disulphide bridges** between cysteine residues on adjacent strands, while enzymic properties depend on the distribution of charged groups.

## Post-translational modification

Post-translational modification includes removal of the N-terminal methionine and cleavage. Association occurs between similar or different polypeptides, or with **prosthetic groups** such as haem.

Polypeptides destined for extracellular secretion are first **glycosylated** in the rough endoplasmic reticulum and Golgi apparatus. Their selection involves a **signal peptide** near the N terminus that binds to a **signal recognition peptide** free in the cytoplasm. This links them to a receptor in the membrane of the endoplasmic reticulum. As it is synthesized the polypeptide is transferred through the membrane; when its carboxyl terminus emerges, the signal peptide is cleaved off. Polypeptides are transported to the Golgi apparatus in vesicles that bud off the endoplasmic reticulum (see Chapter 2).

**Glycosylation** is usually **N linked,** involving addition of a common oligosaccharide to the side chain —NH2 group of asparagine, as in the production of **antibodies** and **lysozymes**. O-linked oligosaccharides are attached to the —OH group on the side chain of serine, threonine or hydroxylysine, as with *secreted* ABO blood group antigens.

Other modifications include **hydroxylation** of lysine and proline, important in creation of the collagen pro-α helix, **sulphation** of tyrosine, as a signal for compartmentalization and **lipidation** of cysteine and glycine residues, necessary for anchoring them to phospholipid membranes. **Acetylation** of lysine in histone H4 modifies its binding to DNA. Protein kinases **phosphorylate** serine and tyrosine residues and can regulate enzymic properties, as in the **proto-oncogene signal transduction cascade** (see Chapter 31).

## Medical issues

**I-cell disease** is due to deficiency in glycosylation of lysozymes. *Ricin* from castor beans blocks EF2; diphtheria toxin blocks translocase.

Many antibiotics target translation specifically **in prokaryotes**. These include *erythromycin* which disrupts translocase, *chloramphenicol*, which interferes with peptidyl transferase, *tetracycline* which prevents binding of aminoacyl tRNAs, *puromycin*, which mimics an aminoacyl tRNA and *streptomycin*, which binds to the small ribosomal subunit. Human mitochondria have an evolutionary affinity with bacteria and some antibiotics interfere with their action.

## The cell cycle

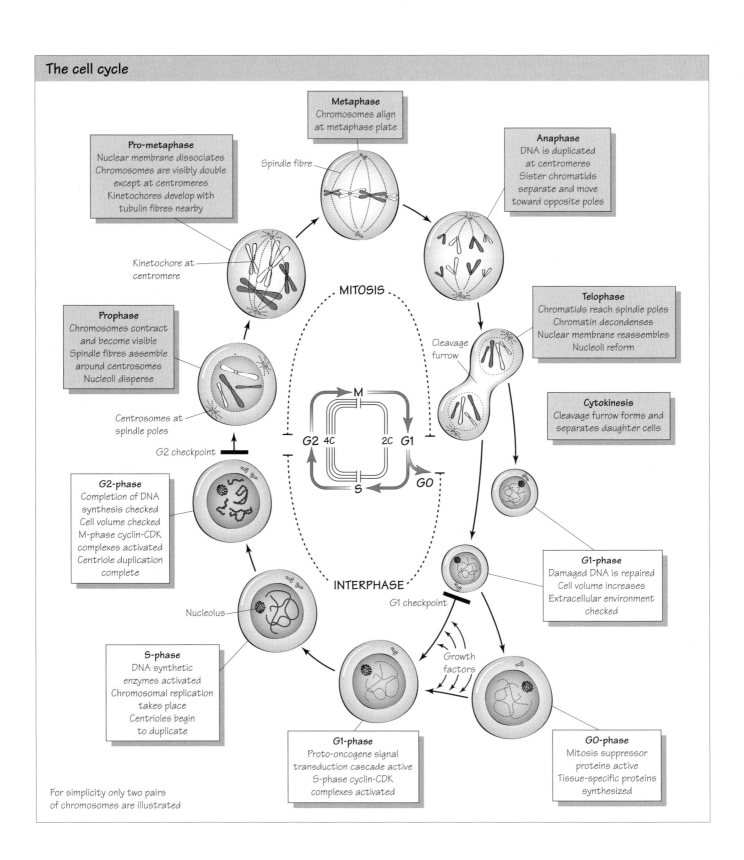

**Metaphase**
Chromosomes align at metaphase plate

**Pro-metaphase**
Nuclear membrane dissociates
Chromosomes are visibly double except at centromeres
Kinetochores develop with tubulin fibres nearby

Spindle fibre

**Anaphase**
DNA is duplicated at centromeres
Sister chromatids separate and move toward opposite poles

Kinetochore at centromere

MITOSIS

**Telophase**
Chromatids reach spindle poles
Chromatin decondenses
Nuclear membrane reassembles
Nucleoli reform

**Prophase**
Chromosomes contract and become visible
Spindle fibres assemble around centrosomes
Nucleoli disperse

Cleavage furrow

**Cytokinesis**
Cleavage furrow forms and separates daughter cells

Centrosomes at spindle poles

M

G2 checkpoint

G2 4C    2C G1

S        G0

**G2-phase**
Completion of DNA synthesis checked
Cell volume checked
M-phase cyclin-CDK complexes activated
Centriole duplication complete

**G1-phase**
Damaged DNA is repaired
Cell volume increases
Extracellular environment checked

INTERPHASE

Nucleolus

G1 checkpoint

**S-phase**
DNA synthetic enzymes activated
Chromosomal replication takes place
Centrioles begin to duplicate

Growth factors

**G1-phase**
Proto-oncogene signal transduction cascade active
S-phase cyclin-CDK complexes activated

**G0-phase**
Mitosis suppressor proteins active
Tissue-specific proteins synthesized

For simplicity only two pairs of chromosomes are illustrated

## Overview

The body grows by increase in cell size and cell number, the latter by division, called **mitosis**. Cells proliferate in response to extracellular **growth factors**, passing through a repeated sequence of events known as **the cell cycle**. This has four major phases: **G1**, then **S**, **G2** and lastly the **mitotic** or **M-phase**. This is followed by division of the cytoplasm and plasma membrane to produce two identical daughter cells. G1, S and G2 together constitute **interphase**. The chromosomes are replicated during the **DNA synthetic** or **S-phase** (see Chapter 5). Most body cells are not actively dividing and are arrested at 'G0' within G1.

Typically the M-phase occupies between a half and one hour of a cycle time of about 20 hours. Normal (as distinct from cancer) human cells can undergo a total of about 80 mitoses, depending on the age of the donor.

## The biochemistry of the cell cycle

The cell cycle is driven by alternating activation and de-activation of key enzymes known as **cyclin-dependent protein kinases (CDKs)**, and their cofactors called **cyclins**. This is performed by phosphorylation and de-phosphorylation by other phosphokinases and phosphatases, specific cyclin-CDK complexes triggering specific phases of the cycle. At appropriate stages the same classes of proteins cause the chromosomes to condense, the nuclear envelope to break down and the microtubules of the cytoskeleton to reorganize to form the mitotic spindle.

## G1-phase

G1 is the gap between M- and S-phases, when the cytoplasm increases in volume. It includes the **G1 checkpoint** when damage to the DNA is repaired and the cell checks that its environment is favourable before committing itself to S-phase. If the nuclear DNA is damaged, a protein called **p53** increases in activity and stimulates transcription of protein **p21**. The latter binds to the specific cyclin-CDK complex responsible for driving the cell into S-phase, so inactivating it and arresting the cell in G1. This allows sufficient time for the DNA repair enzymes to make good the damage to the DNA. If p53 is defective the unrestrained replication that ensues allows that line of cells to accumulate mutations and a cancer can develop. For this reason, p53 is known affectionately as **'the guardian of the genome'**.

## G0-phase

Mammalian cells will proliferate only if stimulated by **extracellular growth factors** secreted by other cells. These operate within the cell through the **proto-oncogene signal transduction cascade** (see Chapter 31). If deprived of such signals during G1, the cell diverts from the cycle and enters the so-called **G0** state. Cells can remain in G0 for years before recommencing division.

The G0 block is imposed by **mitosis-suppressor proteins** such as the **retinoblastoma (Rb) protein** encoded by the *normal* allele of the retinoblastoma gene. These bind to specific regulatory proteins preventing them from stimulating the transcription of genes required for cell proliferation. Extracellular growth factors destroy this block by activating G1-specific cyclin-CDK complexes, which phosphorylate the Rb protein, altering its conformation and causing it to release its bound regulatory proteins. The latter are then free to activate transcription of their target genes and cell proliferation ensues.

## S-phase

The standard number of DNA double-helices per cell, corresponding to the diploid number of single-strand chromosomes, is described as **2C**. The 2C complement is retained throughout G1 and into S-phase, when new chromosomal DNA is synthesized and the cell becomes 4C. From the end of S-phase, through G2 and into M-phase each visually detectable chromosome contains two DNA molecules, known as **sister chromatids**, bound tightly together. In human cells, therefore, from the end of S-phase to the middle of M there are 23 pairs of chromosomes (i.e. 46 observable entities), but 4C (92) nuclear DNA double helices.

Mitosis involves sharing identical sets of chromosomes between the two daughter cells, so that each has 23 pairs and is 2C in terms of its DNA molecules. *G1 and G0 are the only phases of the cell cycle throughout which 46 chromosomes correspond to 2C DNA molecules.*

The replication of DNA during S-phase is described in Chapter 5.

## G2-phase

A second checkpoint on cell size occurs during G2, the gap between S-phase and mitosis. In addition the **G2 checkpoint** allows the cell to check that DNA replication is complete before proceeding to mitosis.

## Mitosis or M-phase

**1 Prophase**. The chromosomes, each consisting of two identical chromatids, begin to contract and become visible within the nucleus. The spindle apparatus of tubulin fibres begins to assemble around the two centrosomes at opposite poles of the cell. The nucleoli disperse.
**2 Pro-metaphase**. The nuclear membrane dissociates. Kinetochores develop around the centromeres of the chromosomes. Tubulin fibres enter the nucleus and assemble radiating out from the kinetochores and linking up with those radiating from the centrosomes.
**3 Metaphase**. Tension in the spindle fibres causes the chromosomes to align midway between the spindle poles, so creating the **metaphase plate**.
**4 Anaphase**. The centromeric DNA shared by sister chromatids is duplicated, they separate and are drawn towards the spindle poles.
**5 Telophase**. The separated sister chromatids (now considered to be chromosomes) reach the spindle poles and a nuclear membrane assembles around each group. The condensed chromatin becomes diffuse and nucleoli reform.
**6 Cytokinesis**. The cell membrane contracts around the mid-region between the poles, creating a **cleavage furrow** which eventually separates the two daughter cells.

## The centrosome cycle

At G1 the pair of centrioles associated with each centrosome separate. During S-phase and G2 a new daughter centriole grows at right angles to each old one. The centrosome then splits at the beginning of M-phase and the two daughter centrosomes move to opposite spindle poles.

## Medical issues

For karyotype analysis (see Chapter 38) dividing cells can be arrested at metaphase with the drug, *colchicine*.

The drug *taxol* prevents spindle disassembly and is used in the treatment of cancer.

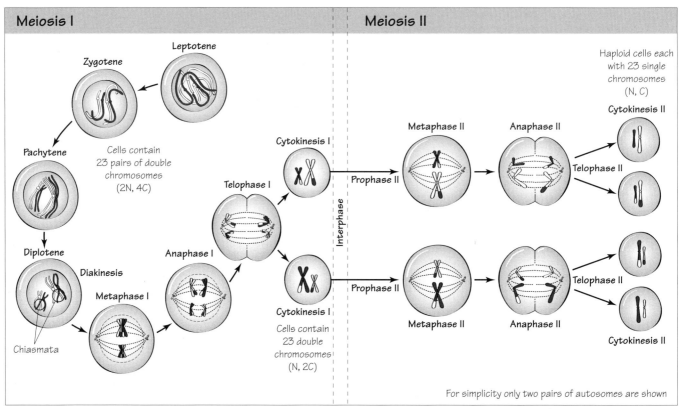

### Meiosis I

Leptotene

Zygotene

Pachytene

Cells contain
23 pairs of double
chromosomes
(2N, 4C)

Diplotene

Diakinesis

Metaphase I

Anaphase I

Telophase I

Cytokinesis I

Chiasmata

Cytokinesis I

Cells contain
23 double
chromosomes
(N, 2C)

Interphase

### Meiosis II

Haploid cells each
with 23 single
chromosomes
(N, C)

Cytokinesis II

Metaphase II

Anaphase II

Telophase II

Prophase II

Prophase II

Metaphase II

Anaphase II

Telophase II

Cytokinesis II

For simplicity only two pairs of autosomes are shown

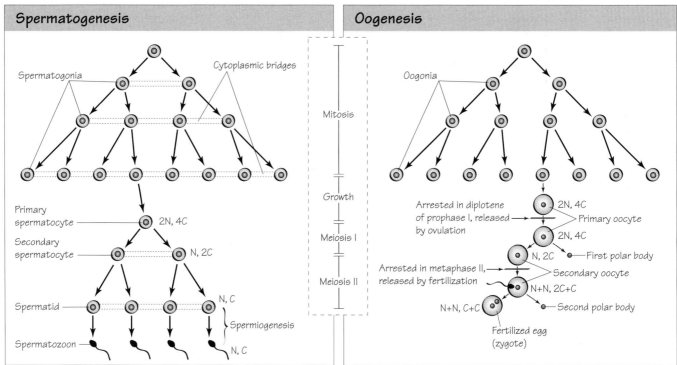

### Spermatogenesis

Spermatogonia

Cytoplasmic bridges

Primary
spermatocyte — 2N, 4C

Secondary
spermatocyte — N, 2C

Spermatid — N, C

Spermatozoon — N, C

Spermiogenesis

### Oogenesis

Oogonia

Mitosis

Growth

Meiosis I

Meiosis II

Arrested in diplotene
of prophase I, released
by ovulation

2N, 4C

2N, 4C — Primary oocyte

N, 2C — First polar body

Arrested in metaphase II,
released by fertilization

Secondary oocyte

N+N, 2C+C

N+N, C+C — Second polar body

Fertilized egg
(zygote)

## Overview

Each body cell contains two sets of chromosomes, one from the mother and one from the father. They are described as 2 N or **diploid**. The sperm and ova contain only one set of chromosomes and are said to be 1 N, or **haploid**. The process by which the diploid number is reduced to haploid during the formation of the germ cells is called **meiosis**. In terms of the number of centromeres, this involves a **reductional division** followed by an **equational division** known as **Meiosis I** and **Meiosis II**. In men meiosis occurs by the pattern seen in most diploid species, but in women there are several differences.

Crossing-over between maternally and paternally derived chromosomes ensures reshuffling of the genetic information between each generation. At **fertilization**, fusion of the haploid chromosome complement of the sperm with that of the ovum restores the chromosome number to diploid in the zygote.

## Meiosis I

Meiosis I has similarities with mitosis, but is much more complex and extended in time. Primary spermatocytes and primary oocytes enter meiosis following G2 of mitosis, so they each have a diploid set of chromosomes (2 N), but each of these contains replicated DNA as **sister chromatids** (i.e. are 4C; see Chapter 9). Prophase I involves reciprocal exchange between maternal and paternal chromatids by the process of **crossing-over**.

## Prophase I

**1 Leptotene**. The chromosomes appear as long threads attached at each end to the nuclear envelope.

**2 Zygotene**. The chromosomes contract, pair with and adhere closely to (or '**synapse** with') their homologues. This normally involves precise registration, gene for gene throughout the entire genome. In primary spermatocytes X- and Y-chromosomes synapse at the tips of their short arms only.

**3 Pachytene**. Sister chromatids begin to separate, the double chromosome being known as a **bivalent**. The chromosome pair represented by four double helices is called a **tetrad**. One or both chromatids of each paternal chromosome crosses over with those from the mother in what is known as **synaptonemal complex**. Every chromosome pair undergoes at least one cross-over.

**4 Diplotene**. The chromatids separate except at the regions of cross-over or **chiasmata** (singular: **chiasma**). This situation persists in all **primary oocytes** until they are shed at **ovulation**.

**5 Diakinesis**. the reorganized chromosomes begin to move apart. Each bivalent can now be seen to contain four chromatids linked by a common centromere, while non-sister chromatids are linked by chiasmata.

**Metaphase I, Anaphase I, Telophase I, Cytokinesis I**. These follow a similar course to the equivalent stages in mitosis (see Chapter 9), the critical difference being that, instead of non-sister chromatids being segregated, pairs of reciprocally crossed-over sister chromatids joined at their centromeres are distributed to the daughter cells.

At the end of Meiosis I, secondary spermatocytes and secondary oocytes contain 23 chromosomes (1 N), each consisting of two chromatids (i.e. 2C).

## Meiosis II

There is a transient interphase, during which no chromosome replication occurs, followed by prophase, metaphase, anaphase, telophase and cytokinesis. These resemble the equivalent phases of mitosis in that pairs of chromatids (bivalents) linked at their centromeres become aligned at the metaphase plate and are then drawn into separate daughter cells following replication of the centromeric DNA.

At the end of Meiosis II the cells contain 23 chromosomes (1 N), each consisting of a single chromatid (1C).

## Male meiosis

Spermatogenesis includes all the events by which spermatogonia are transformed into spermatozoa and takes about 64 days. Cytokinesis is incomplete throughout, so that each generation of cells remains linked by cytoplasmic bridges.

A diploid **primary spermatocyte** undergoes Meiosis I to form two haploid **secondary spermatocytes**. These both undergo Meiosis II to produce four haploid **spermatids**. The spermatids become elaborated into **spermatozoa** during **spermiogenesis**. This includes: (i) formation of the acrosome containing enzymes that assist with penetration of the egg; (ii) condensation of the nucleus; (iii) shedding of most of the cytoplasm; and (iv) formation of the neck, midpiece and tail.

## Female meiosis

Oogenesis begins in the fetus at 12 weeks, but ceases abruptly at about 20 weeks, the **primary oocytes** remaining at diplotene of prophase I until ovulation, this suspended state being called **dictyotene**.

Ovulation begins at puberty and usually only one oocyte is shed per month. Under stimulation by hormones a primary oocyte swells accumulating cytoplasmic materials. At completion of Meiosis I these are inherited by one daughter cell, the **secondary oocyte**. The other nucleus passes into the **first polar body**, which usually degenerates without further division. Meiosis I is completed rapidly then, after a pause, the secondary oocyte is shed into the uterine, or Fallopian, tube.

Meiosis II stops at metaphase until the entry of a sperm. It then completes division, producing a large haploid **ovum** pro-nucleus, which fuses with the sperm pro-nucleus, and a very small **second polar body**, which degenerates.

The whole process takes from 12 to 50 years, depending when fertilization takes place.

## The significance of meiosis

**1** The diploid chromosome content of somatic cells is reduced to haploid in the gametes.

**2** Paternal and maternal chromosomes become reassorted, with a potential for $2^{23}$ ($= 8\,388\,608$) different combinations, excluding recombination *within* chromosomes.

**3** Reassortment of paternal and maternal alleles *within* chromosomes creates an infinite potential for genetic variation between gametes.

**4** The *randomness* of reassortment of paternal and maternal alleles during meiosis (and at fertilization) ensures the applicability of probability theory to genetic ratios and the general validity of Mendel's laws (see Chapter 16).

**5** The frequency of cross-over between genes *within* chromosomes allows the relative positions of genes to be mapped (see Chapters 27, 28).

**6** Errors sometimes occur at chromosome pairing and crossing-over, which can produce **translocations**, as well as at their separation or **disjunction**, which can lead to **aneuploidy** (see Chapter 14).

## Fertilization and implantation (uterus not to scale)

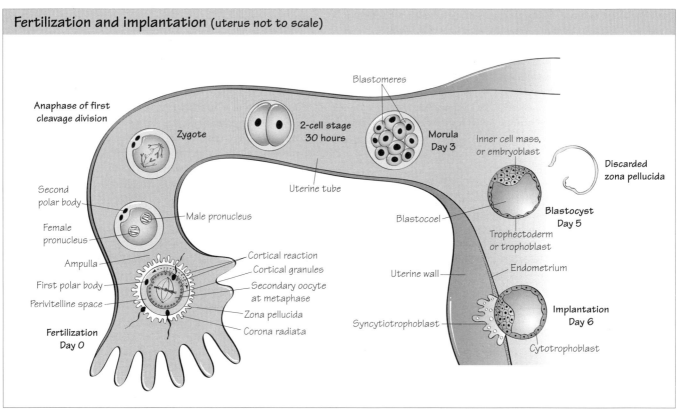

Anaphase of first cleavage division

Zygote

2-cell stage 30 hours

Blastomeres

Morula Day 3

Inner cell mass, or embryoblast

Discarded zona pellucida

Second polar body

Female pronucleus

Male pronucleus

Ampulla

First polar body

Perivitelline space

Fertilization Day 0

Uterine tube

Cortical reaction

Cortical granules

Secondary oocyte at metaphase

Zona pellucida

Corona radiata

Blastocoel

Uterine wall

Syncytiotrophoblast

Blastocyst Day 5

Trophectoderm or trophoblast

Endometrium

Implantation Day 6

Cytotrophoblast

## Formation of the embryonic disc

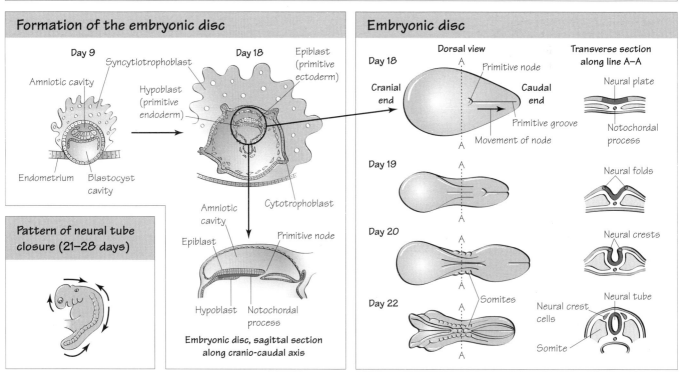

Day 9

Amniotic cavity

Syncytiotrophoblast

Hypoblast (primitive endoderm)

Day 18

Epiblast (primitive ectoderm)

Endometrium

Blastocyst cavity

Amniotic cavity

Cytotrophoblast

Epiblast

Primitive node

Hypoblast

Notochordal process

Embryonic disc, sagittal section along cranio-caudal axis

### Pattern of neural tube closure (21–28 days)

## Embryonic disc

Day 18

Dorsal view

Transverse section along line A–A

Cranial end

Primitive node

Caudal end

Neural plate

Primitive groove

Movement of node

Notochordal process

Day 19

Neural folds

Day 20

Neural crests

Day 22

Somites

Neural crest cells

Neural tube

Somite

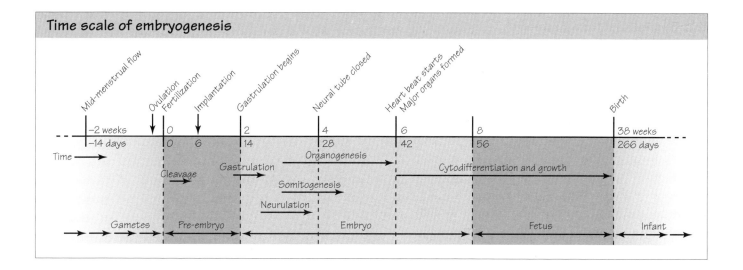

## Time scale of embryogenesis

## Overview

**Fertilization** by a sperm initiates **embryogenesis**. Mitosis ensues and the **pre-embryo** implants in the uterus. The **embryo** proper develops from a few internal cells, through creation of three **embryonic germ layers**. **Organogenesis** involves interactions between these and is completed by 6–8 weeks. During the subsequent period of **growth** and **cytodifferentiation** the individual is called a **fetus**.

## The pre-embryo (days 0–14)

The secondary oocyte is shed into the peritoneal cavity and directed into the adjacent **uterine** (Fallopian) **tube**, where fertilization must take place within 24 hours. The sperm performs four functions: (i) *stimulation of metaphase II in the secondary oocyte*; (ii) *restoration of the diploid number of chromosomes*; (iii) *initiation of cleavage*; and (iv) *determination of sex*.

The sperm passes through the **corona cells** on the oocyte surface and adheres to the **zona pellucida**. The **acrosome** in the sperm head then releases enzymes that digest a tunnel through the zona pellucida, allowing the sperm to pass into the **perivitelline space** and fuse with the oocyte membrane. The sperm head becomes engulfed by the oocyte, entry of more sperms being prevented by a rapid **cortical reaction**. The oocyte nucleus completes metaphase II, expels the second polar body and maternal and paternal **pronuclei** fuse to form the **zygote**.

Mitosis of the pre-embryo is called **cleavage**, and the resultant **blastomeres** are smaller after each division, the 16-cell **morula** passing down the uterine tube aided by peristalsis and ciliary movement. A space called the **blastocoel** forms off-centre in the morula to create the **blastocyst**, which swells and bursts from the zona pellucida. Two different cell types are now recognizable: the flattened **trophectoderm** cells of the outer **trophoblast** and the eccentrically placed **inner cell mass** or **embryoblast**.

On day 6 the blastocyst implants in the endometrium lining the uterus. Some trophoblast cells fuse to form the invasive **syncytiotrophoblast**, the remainder constituting the **cytotrophoblast**. The blastocyst now takes nourishment from the mother and grows rapidly as it sinks further into the endometrium.

The inner cell mass exposed ventrally to the blastocoel flattens to form the **primitive endoderm,** or **hypoblast**, while the remainder forms the **primitive ectoderm,** or **epiblast**, within which develops the **amniotic cavity**. A double-layered disc called the **embryonic disc** forms from the epiblast and hypoblast at 7–12 days, *from which the embryo proper develops*.

## The embryo (weeks 2–8)

**Gastrulation** is the process which creates the **embryonic mesoderm** and initiates activity of the embryo's own genes. The **primitive streak** first appears in the epiblast at the caudal (tail) end of the embryonic disc, extends towards its centre and then develops the **primitive groove** in its amniotic (i.e. dorsal) surface. At the cranial (head) end of this develops a nodule of cells called the **primitive** (or **Hensen's**) **node**.

Epiblast cells migrate across the disc, through the primitive groove and into the space above the hypoblast. These become the embryonic mesoderm, creating the three **germ layers**: ectoderm from the epiblast, **mesoderm** and **endoderm** from the hypoblast together with some epiblast cells that merge with it. Mesoderm cells that migrate anteriorly and accumulate in the midline form the **notochordal process**, which later extends caudally.

The epiblast thickens to form the **neural plate** and a **neural fold** arises on either side of the central axis. These curve over, contact and from 22 days fuse in five separate movements to create the **neural tube**, which later becomes the spinal cord. Along the dorsal edges of the neural folds are the **neural crest cells** that migrate out to give rise to several cell types, including nerve, bone, supporting structures of the heart, adrenalin-secreting and pigment cells. As the primitive node moves caudally down the midline, blocks of mesoderm on either side rotate to create 42–44 pairs of segmental **somites**, the most caudal 5–7 of which subsequently disappear.

## The fetus (weeks 8–38)

The ectoderm is the origin of the outer epithelium and CNS and, with mesoderm, peripheral structures such as limbs; mesoderm forms muscles, circulatory system, kidneys, sex organs and together with endoderm, the internal organs; endoderm gives rise to the gut and digestive glands. The rudiments of all the major organs are formed through 'inductive' tissue interactions by about 6 weeks, when the heart starts beating. Thereafter development mainly involves increase in the number and types of cells. Birth normally occurs at 38 weeks.

# 12 Sexual differentiation

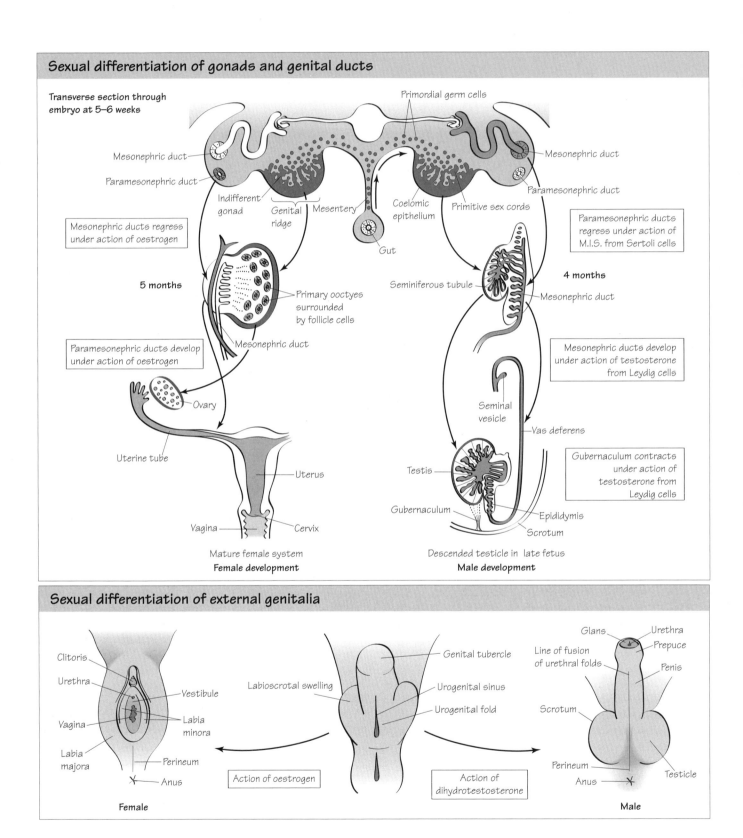

## Sexual differentiation of gonads and genital ducts

Transverse section through embryo at 5–6 weeks

Primordial germ cells

Mesonephric duct
Paramesonephric duct
Indifferent gonad
Genital ridge
Mesentery
Coelomic epithelium
Gut
Primitive sex cords
Mesonephric duct
Paramesonephric duct

Mesonephric ducts regress under action of oestrogen

Paramesonephric ducts regress under action of M.I.S. from Sertoli cells

5 months

4 months

Seminiferous tubule
Mesonephric duct

Primary ooctyes surrounded by follicle cells
Mesonephric duct

Paramesonephric ducts develop under action of oestrogen

Mesonephric ducts develop under action of testosterone from Leydig cells

Ovary

Seminal vesicle
Vas deferens

Uterine tube

Gubernaculum contracts under action of testosterone from Leydig cells

Uterus

Testis

Vagina
Cervix

Gubernaculum
Epididymis
Scrotum

Mature female system
**Female development**

Descended testicle in late fetus
**Male development**

## Sexual differentiation of external genitalia

Clitoris
Urethra
Vestibule
Vagina
Labia minora
Labia majora
Perineum
Anus

Genital tubercle
Labioscrotal swelling
Urogenital sinus
Urogenital fold

Action of oestrogen

Action of dihydrotestosterone

Glans
Urethra
Prepuce
Line of fusion of urethral folds
Penis
Scrotum
Perineum
Anus
Testicle

**Female**

**Male**

## Overview

Sexual differentiation is initiated at fertilization, depending on whether the sperm carries an X or a Y chromosome. At the blastocyst stage in XX embryos one X chromosome in every cell is permanently inactivated, otherwise development of the sexes is similar until the **SRY gene** on the Y chromosome comes into operation and certain structures, including the brain, become progressively more masculinized.

## X chromosome inactivation

At the late blastocyst stage cells inactivate all but one of their X chromosomes. The nuclei of normal XX female cells therefore come to contain one inactive X, which can be seen at interphase as a Barr body in addition to their active X (see Chapter 20). Presence or absence of a **Barr body** is the basis of the original Olympic sex test. The choice of whether it is the paternal, or maternal X which becomes inactive is random in each somatic cell, but in descendent cells it remains the same. Every woman therefore develops as a mosaic with respect to expression of her two X chromosomes. In the extra-embryonic trophoblast cells the paternal X is preferentially inactivated. In oogonia the inactive chromosome is reactivated.

Genes in the pairing (**pseudo-autosomal**) region and several other sites on the X are not subject to inactivation, accounting for the sexual abnormalities of XXY and XO individuals (see Chapter 14).

## Early development

At the beginning of week 5, up to 2000 **primordial germ cells** migrate from the endoderm cells of the yolk sac and infiltrate the **primitive sex cords** within the mesodermal **genital ridges**, which are developments of the coelomic epithelium. The paired **indifferent gonad** is identical in males and females.

## The ovary

In the early ovary the primitive sex cords break down, but the surface epithelium proliferates and gives rise to the **cortical cords**, which split into clusters, each surrounding one or more germ cells. The latter, now called **oogonia**, proliferate then enter meiosis as **primary oocytes**.

## The testis

The SRY gene carried only on the Y chromosome is expressed in week 7 in the cells of the primitive sex cords. Its product is a **zinc finger protein** (a gene switching protein) that binds to DNA in those same cells, leading to a new pattern of specific gene expression. These cells proliferate into the **testis cords**.

**Leydig cells** derived from the original mesenchyme of the gonadal ridge move in around the 8th week and until weeks 17–18 synthesize male sex hormones, or **androgens**, including **testosterone**, which initiate sexual differentiation of the genital ducts and external genitalia. By the 4th month the male gonads also contain **Sertoli cells** derived from the surface epithelium of the gonad.

## Genital ducts

Initially both sexes have two pairs of genital ducts: **mesonephric** (or **Wolffian**) and **paramesonephric** (or **Müllerian**). In females the mesonephric ducts regress under the action of **oestrogens** produced by the maternal system, placenta and fetal ovaries, but the paramesonephric ducts remain and become the **uterine tubes** and **uterus**.

In males the Sertoli cells produce a growth factor called **Müllerian inhibiting substance** (**MIS**), which causes the paramesonephric ducts to degenerate.

Testosterone binds to an intracellular receptor protein and the hormone-receptor complex then binds to specific control sites in the DNA and regulates transcription of tissue-specific genes. In male embryos testosterone converts the mesonephric ducts into the **vas deferens** and **epididymis**.

## External genitalia

The external genitalia are derived from a complex of mesodermal tissue located around the **urogenital sinus**. At the end of the 6th week in both sexes this consists of the **genital tubercle** anteriorly, the paired **urogenital folds** on either side and lateral to these the **labioscrotal swellings**.

In females oestrogen stimulates slight elongation of the genital tubercle to form the **clitoris**, while the urogenital folds remain separate as the **labia minora**. The urogenital sinus remains open as the **vestibule** and the labioscrotal swellings become the **labia majora**.

The tissues around the **urogenital sinus** synthesize **5-alpha-reductase** which in males converts **testosterone** secreted by the Leydig cells to **dihydrotestosterone**. Under the action of this hormone the genital tubercle elongates into the **penis**, pulling the urethral folds forward to form the lateral walls of the **urethral groove**. At the end of the 3rd month the tops of the walls fuse to create the **penile urethra**, while the urogenital sinus becomes the **prostate**.

## Descent of the testis

Usually in the 7th month the testes descend from the peritoneal cavity between the peritoneal epithelium and pubic bones and into the **scrotum**. This is mediated finally by the **gubernaculum** contracting under the influence of testosterone, but descent may not be completed until birth.

## Puberty

Puberty is triggered by hormones secreted by the **pituitary gland** acting on ovaries, testes and adrenal glands. In girls, usually between ages 10 and 14, the ovaries respond by secreting oestrogen that stimulates breast growth. About a year later menstruation commences, accompanied by maturation of the uterus and vagina and broadening of the pelvis. Testosterone synthesis is stimulated in the adrenal glands and is responsible for growth of pubic and axillary (underarm) hair in girls.

In boys, starting at about 11–12 years, the testes enlarge and synthesis of androgens is reactivated. The testis cords acquire a lumen, so forming the **seminiferous tubules**, which link up with the urethra. The androgens enhance growth of the penis and larynx and initiate spermatogenesis.

## Medical issues

The most common causes of ambiguous genitalia are **adrenal hyperplasia** in girls and **androgen insufficiency** in boys. Patients with **testicular feminization syndrome** inherit a Y chromosome, but develop a convincing female external phenotype because they lack testosterone receptors. Failure of testicular descent is called **cryptorchidism**.

Tumours arising from primordial germ cells are known as **teratomas**. They can contain several well-differentiated tissues (e.g. hair, bone, sebaceous gland, thyroid tissue) and are usually benign (see Chapter 31).

# 13 The place of genetics in medicine

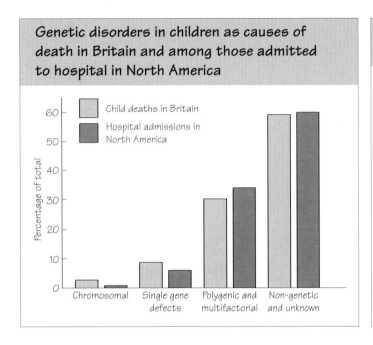

**Genetic disorders in children as causes of death in Britain and among those admitted to hospital in North America**

- Child deaths in Britain
- Hospital admissions in North America

Percentage of total

Chromosomal | Single gene defects | Polygenic and multifactorial | Non-genetic and unknown

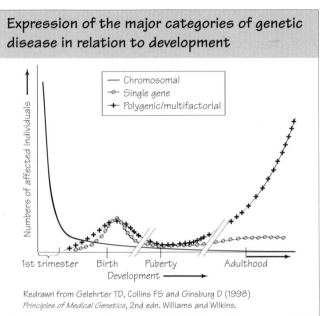

**Expression of the major categories of genetic disease in relation to development**

- Chromosomal
- Single gene
- Polygenic/multifactorial

Numbers of affected individuals

1st trimester | Birth | Puberty | Adulthood

Development ⟶

Redrawn from Gelehrter TD, Collins FS and Ginsburg D (1998) *Principles of Medical Genetics*, 2nd edn. Williams and Wilkins.

## Introduction

The true scale of genetic disease has only recently become appreciated. One survey of over a million consecutive births showed that at least one in 20 people under the age of 25 develop a serious disease with a major genetic component. This, however, is probably an underestimate as it depends on how disease is defined and how strong the genetic component needs to be for it to be included.

Studies of the causes of death of more than 1200 British children suggest that about 40% died as a result of a genetic condition. Other studies in North America indicate that genetic factors are important in 50% of the admissions to paediatric (children's) hospitals. Through variation in immune responsiveness, genetic factors even play a role in infectious diseases, although these might be thought to be wholly environmental.

Traditionally genetic diseases are classified into three major categories: **chromosomal**, **single gene** and **multifactorial**. Chromosomal defects can create major physiological disruption and most are incompatible with even prenatal survival. These are responsible for the vast majority of deaths in the first trimester of pregnancy and about 2.5% of childhood deaths. Most single-gene defects reveal their presence after birth and are responsible for 6–9% of early **morbidity** (sickness) and mortality. The multifactorial disorders account for about 30% of childhood illness and in middle-to-late adult life play a major role in the common illnesses from which most of us will die.

## Overview of Part II

### Chromosomal defects (Chapters 14 and 15)

If chromosome segregation is incomplete or unequal at meiosis, chromosomally abnormal embryos can result. Since an average chromosome carries about 2000 genes, too many or too few chromosomes cause gross abnormalities of phenotype, most of which are incompat-ible with survival. Abnormal or unequal exchange of chromosomal material creates a variety of abnormalities, of varying severity. These are described in Chapters 14 and 15. It is interesting to note that the three chromosomes associated with live birth of chromosomal triomies (13, 18 and 21) are the ones with the lowest gene density or the smallest size.

### Single gene defects (Chapters 16–19)

The foundation of the science of genetics is a set of principles of heredity discovered in the mid-19th century by an Augustinian monk called Gregor Mendel and described in Chapter 16. These give rise to characteristic patterns of inheritance, depending on whether the disease is dominant or recessive. Recognition of the pattern of inheritance of a disease is central to prediction of the risk of producing an affected child, as described in Chapters 17 and 18. Chapter 18 also explains the risks associated with consanguineous mating. Chapter 19 deals with single-gene conditions that are less easily classified.

### Sex-related inheritance (Chapter 20)

There are many reasons why the sexes may express diseases differently. Of these the most important relates to the possession by males of only a single X-chromosome. Most sex-related inherited disease involves expression in males of recessive alleles carried on the X. The most common conditions in this category are defective colour vision and neurodevelopmental delay (mental retardation) in males. Mitochondrial disorders are uniquely transmitted by mothers to all their children.

### Congenital and complex traits (Chapters 21–24)

Some conditions, including many congenital abnormalities, are due to the combined action of several genes, or the adverse effects of environmental factors. These fall into the category of multifactorial inheritance. Genetic counselling in relation to this group is generally problematic as patterns of inheritance are usually not discernible. Multifactorial traits are of immense importance as they include most of the common disorders of adult life. Much current research is concentrated in this area.

## Polymorphism (Chapters 25 and 26)

'Polymorphism' refers to variation between normally healthy individuals. This concept is especially important in **pharmacogenetics**, blood transfusion and organ transplantation. The frequency of polymorphisms within populations is dealt with in Chapter 26.

## Genetic linkage and association (Chapters 27 and 28)

If genes reside side-by-side on the same chromosome they are 'genetically linked'. If one is a disease gene, but cannot easily be detected whereas its neighbour can, then alleles of the latter can be used as markers for the disease allele. This allows prenatal assessment, informing decisions about pregnancy termination, selection of embryos fertilized *in vitro,* presymptomatic diagnosis and diagnosis of problematic conditions.

'Genetic association' refers to the coincident presence of certain alleles with certain diseases although the basis of the relationship may be obscure.

## Mutation and its consequences (Chapters 29–32)

Mutation of DNA can involve chemical modification of bases, destruction, deletion or relocation of critical sequences. Repair mechanisms usually correct much of the damage, but new alleles are sometimes created that can be passed on to offspring. It is generally accepted that most mutational changes are either neutral in effect or deleterious, although very, very occasionally a new, apparently beneficial allele does appear. Geneticists therefore generally consider that conditions which increase the rate of mutation are best avoided.

Damage that occurs to the DNA of somatic cells can result in cancer, when a cell starts to proliferate out of control. This can give rise to a tumour which may break up and its component cells migrate and establish secondary tumours. The molecular details of **carcinogenesis** are outlined in Chapter 31 and families with a tendency toward cancer are described in Chapter 32.

## Immunogenetics (Chapter 33)

A healthy immune system may eliminate many thousands of potential cancer cells every day, in addition to disposing of infectious organisms. Molecular biologists believe that the genetic events that take place in the immune system are unique to that system. These events involve cutting, splicing and reassembly of alternative DNA sequences to create billions of new genes within individual B- and T-lymphocytes. An outline of these events is given in Chapter 33.

# 14 Chromosomal aneuploidies

## Down syndrome

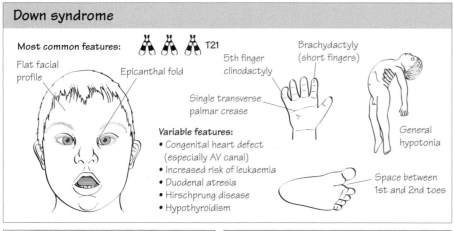

**Most common features:** T21

Flat facial profile

Epicanthal fold

5th finger clinodactyly

Brachydactyly (short fingers)

Single transverse palmar crease

General hypotonia

**Variable features:**
• Congenital heart defect (especially AV canal)
• Increased risk of leukaemia
• Duodenal atresia
• Hirschprung disease
• Hypothyroidism

Space between 1st and 2nd toes

## Edward syndrome

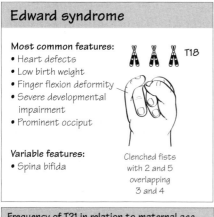

**Most common features:**
• Heart defects
• Low birth weight
• Finger flexion deformity
• Severe developmental impairment
• Prominent occiput

T18

**Variable features:**
• Spina bifida

Clenched fists with 2 and 5 overlapping 3 and 4

## Patau syndrome

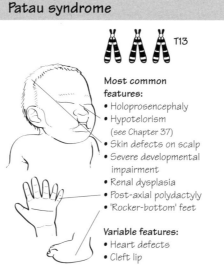

T13

**Most common features:**
• Holoprosencephaly
• Hypotelorism (see Chapter 37)
• Skin defects on scalp
• Severe developmental impairment
• Renal dysplasia
• Post-axial polydactyly
• 'Rocker-bottom' feet

**Variable features:**
• Heart defects
• Cleft lip

## Turner syndrome

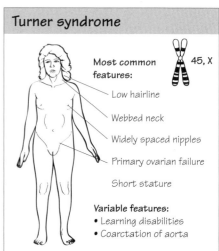

**Most common features:**

45, X

Low hairline

Webbed neck

Widely spaced nipples

Primary ovarian failure

Short stature

**Variable features:**
• Learning disabilities
• Coarctation of aorta

## Klinefelter syndrome

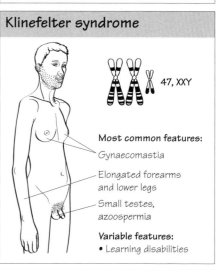

47, XXY

**Most common features:**

Gynaecomastia

Elongated forearms and lower legs

Small testes, azoospermia

**Variable features:**
• Learning disabilities

## Frequency of T21 in relation to maternal age, diagnosis by amniocentesis and at birth

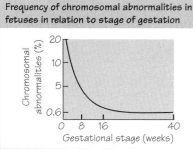

Amniocentesis

Birth

T21 frequency (%)

Maternal age (years)

## Frequency of chromosomal abnormalities in fetuses in relation to stage of gestation

Chromosomal abnormalities (%)

Gestational stage (weeks)

## Causation of chromosomal aneuploidies

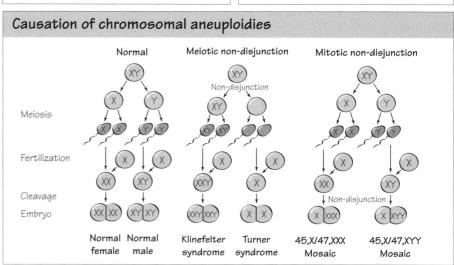

Normal    Meiotic non-disjunction    Mitotic non-disjunction

Meiosis

Non-disjunction

Fertilization

Cleavage

Embryo

Non-disjunction

Normal female   Normal male   Klinefelter syndrome   Turner syndrome   45,X/47,XXX Mosaic   45,X/47,XYY Mosaic

## Overview

Chromosomal disorders involve both abnormal numbers of chromosomes and aberrations in their structure (see Chapter 15). **Euploidy** means that the chromosome number per body cell is an integral multiple of the haploid number, $N = 23$, **aneuploidy** that it is other than an integral multiple. **Diploidy** describes the normal situation, a typical body cell in humans having $2N = 46$ chromosomes. Women have 23 similar pairs, including a pair of X chromosomes, their **karyotype** formula being **46,XX**. In normal men there is an X and a Y chromosome, their karyotype being **46,XY**. **Polyploidy** refers to multiples of the haploid number (e.g. **triploidy**, $3N = 69$).

**Trisomy** $(2N + 1)$ refers to the presence of three copies of one chromosome. Possession of only a single copy of an autosome $(2N - 1)$ is called **monosomy**.

**Mosaic** individuals contain two different cell lines derived from one zygote. A **chimaera** also contains two different cell lines, but is derived by fusion of two zygotes (e.g. a 46,XX/46,XY **hermaphrodite**).

Possibly as many as 25% of conceptions involve a chromosomal disorder, but this is reduced to 0.6% at birth by natural loss, mainly during the first trimester.

The non-sex chromosomes are called **autosomes**. Trisomies 21, 18 and 13 are the only autosomal trisomies compatible with survival to birth and only Trisomy 21 with life beyond infancy.

## Down syndrome, Trisomy 21

**1 Karyotype**. Trisomy 21 (**47,XX,+21** or **47,XY,+21**) accounts for about 96% of cases of Down syndrome. The remaining 4% have translocations between 21 and another chromosome (see Chapters 15 and 29). Some patients are **mosaics.**

**2 Incidence**. About 1/700 live births.

**3 Features**. Typically there are **epicanthal folds** and a flat, broad face. Other features include a large gap between first and second toes, webbing of toes 2 and 3, general **hypotonia** (poor muscle tone), flat **occiput** (back of skull), short stature, **Brushfield spots** in irides, **single transverse crease** in the palm, single fold on and **clinodactyly** of fifth digit (see figure), open mouth with protruding tongue that lacks a central fissure, hearing deficit (60–80%), increased risk of infection, **leukaemia** (80%), congenital heart defects (40–50%) and **epilepsy** (5–10%). IQ is 25–75, with typically a happy temperament, but Alzheimer-like dementia may occur in up to 50% in mid-life and there is often early-onset **atheromatous** (i.e. with fatty deposits) degeneration of the cardiovascular system, **Hirschprung disease** and **hypothyroidism** (15–20%).

**4 Life expectancy**. Due to heart defects, for some it is less than 50 years.

## Edward syndrome, Trisomy 18

**1 Karyotype**. **47,XX,+18** or **47,XY,+18**.

**2 Incidence**. About 1/3000 live births.

**3 Features**. Clenched fists with index and fifth fingers overlapping the rest; 'rocker bottom' feet with prominent heels; low-set, malformed ears; micrognathia (small lower jaw); single palmar crease; growth deficiency; cardiac and renal abnormalities; prominent occiput and general hypotonia.

**4 Mean survival time**. About 2 months; 30% die within a month; only 10% survive beyond a year.

## Patau syndrome, Trisomy 13

**1 Karyotype**. **47,XX,+13** or **47,XY,+13**.

**2 Incidence**. About 1/5000 live births.

**3 Features**. Microcephaly (small head) with sloping forehead; holoprosencephaly (failure of formation of paired cerebral hemispheres); 'rocker-bottom' feet, microphthalmia, anophthalmia, cyclopia or hypotelorism (i.e. small or absent eyes, a single central eye or closely spaced eyes); cryptorchidism (undescended testicles); simian crease; heart defects; cleft lip and palate; micrognathia and postaxial polydactyly (sixth finger present).

**4 Survival rate**. Similar to Edward syndrome, with rather more (50%) dying within the first month.

## Klinefelter syndrome

**1 Karyotype**. **47,XXY** (or **48,XXXY**; **49,XXXXY**, etc.).

**2 Incidence**. About 1/500 male births.

**3 Features**. Phenotype is basically male, but with **gynaecomastia** (breasts) and feminine body hair distribution (but masculine facial hair); small genitalia and infertility. They are tall, with elongated lower legs and forearms. There may be learning difficulties, **scoliosis** (spinal curvature), **emphysema** (gaseous distension of lung tissues), **osteoporosis** (skeletal breakdown) and **varicose veins**; 8% have **diabetes mellitus**.

## Turner syndrome

**1 Karyotype**. **45,X**.

**2 Incidence**. 1/5000 female births. (The fetus aborts in over 95% of cases.)

**3 Features**. Phenotype is basically female, but patients fail to mature sexually. There is often also **lymphoedema** (excess fluid) in the hands and feet of newborns; excess skin forming a web between neck and shoulders and low posterior hairline; heart-shaped face with micrognathia, epicanthal folds and **strabismus** (squint); short stature; short fourth metacarpals; many **naevi** (moles), shield-shaped chest with widely spaced nipples; increased 'carrying angle' at elbow (**cubitus valgus**). Intelligence is normal. There is congenital heart disease in 20%, unexplained **hypertension** (high blood pressure) in 30%, kidney malformations and **thyroiditis**. They may develop X-linked recessive disease as in males. Some Turner syndrome patients are mosaics (45,X; 46,XY).

## XYY syndrome

**1 Karyotype**. **47,XYY**.

**2 Incidence**. 1/1000 male births.

**3 Features**. Very tall stature, large teeth, learning disabilities, sometimes problems in motor coordination. Early claims of predisposition to aggressive behaviour are not generally upheld. Fertility is normal.

## Triple X syndrome

**1 Karyotype**. **47,XXX**.

**2 Incidence**. 1/1000 female births

**3 Features**. Generally tall with some learning problems and difficulty in interpersonal relationships. Claims of reduced fertility are now sometimes ascribed to 45,X oocytes in 45,X/47,XXX mosaics.

## Causation

**Aneuploidy** is usually ascribed to **failure of conjugation** of chromosomes in meiosis I; or **non-disjunction**, **premature disjunction** or **anaphase lag** (delayed separation) in meiosis II. The frequency of chromosomal errors in oocytes increases dramatically with *maternal age* (see figure). **Mosaics** can be caused by chromosomal non-disjunction during *mitosis*.

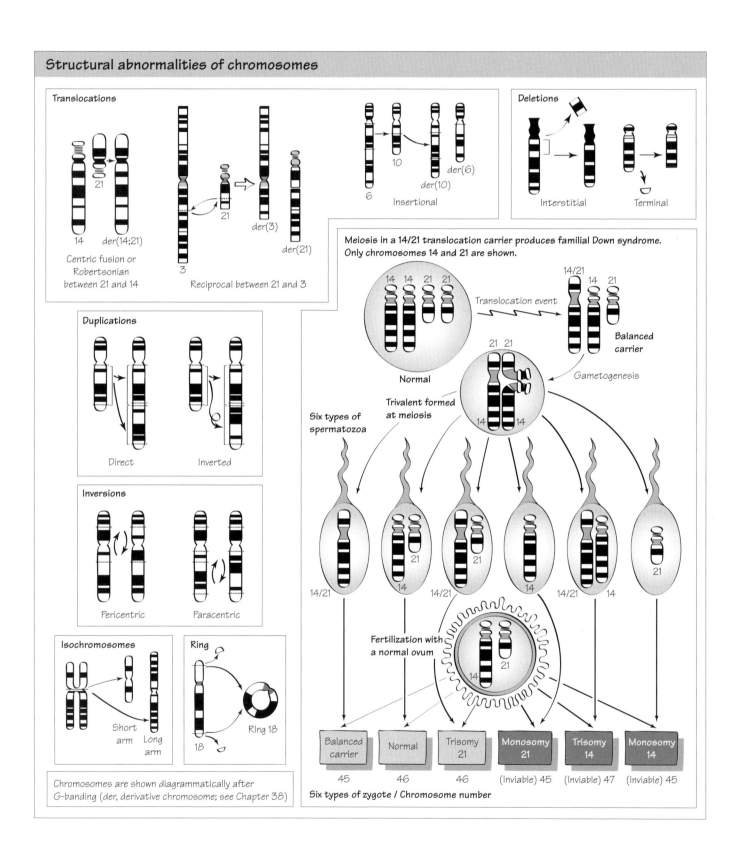

Structural abnormalities of chromosomes

**Translocations**

14    der(14;21)

Centric fusion or
Robertsonian
between 21 and 14

21

3    der(3)
    der(21)

Reciprocal between 21 and 3

6    10    der(10)    der(6)

Insertional

**Deletions**

Interstitial    Terminal

**Duplications**

Direct    Inverted

**Inversions**

Pericentric    Paracentric

**Isochromosomes**

Short
arm    Long
arm

**Ring**

18    Ring 18

Chromosomes are shown diagrammatically after
G-banding (der, derivative chromosome; see Chapter 38)

Meiosis in a 14/21 translocation carrier produces familial Down syndrome.
Only chromosomes 14 and 21 are shown.

14  14  21  21

Normal

Translocation event

14/21  14  21

Balanced
carrier

21  21

Trivalent formed
at meiosis

14  14

Gametogenesis

Six types of
spermatozoa

14/21    14    14/21    14    14/21    14    21
    21    21

Fertilization with
a normal ovum

14    21

| Balanced carrier | Normal | Trisomy 21 | Monosomy 21 | Trisomy 14 | Monosomy 14 |
|---|---|---|---|---|---|
| 45 | 46 | 46 | (Inviable) 45 | (Inviable) 47 | (Inviable) 45 |

Six types of zygote / Chromosome number

## Overview

Structural aberrations include **translocations, deletions, ring chromosomes, duplications, inversions, isochromosomes** and **centric fragments**. Most of these result from unequal exchange between homologous repeated sequences on the same or different chromosomes, or when two chromosome breaks occur close together and enzymic repair mechanisms link the wrong ends.

## Translocations

A translocation involves exchange of chromosomal material between chromosomes. Three types are recognized: **centric fusion** or '**Robertsonian**', **reciprocal** and **insertional**.

### Centric fusion or 'Robertsonian' translocations

Centric fusion arises from breaks at or near the centromeres of two chromosomes, followed by their fusion. The long arms of chromosomes 13, 14, 15, 21 and 22 are most commonly involved, especially 13 with 14, and 14 with 21. These are all **acrocentric** chromosomes with very small short arms (see Chapter 38), the latter carrying multiple copies of the ribosomal RNA genes (see Chapter 6).

Although centric fusion involves loss of rRNA genes, sufficient intact copies remain for no serious consequence to result. The carrier of a pair of centrically fused chromosomes may therefore have only 45 chromosomes, but be quite healthy as the overall loss is insignificant. This is a **balanced translocation**.

When centrically fused chromosomes pair during meiosis a **trivalent** structure is formed allowing contact between homologous chromosome segments. At anaphase six possible gametic combinations can then be formed: one normal, one abnormal but balanced and four unbalanced (see figure). However, selection of gametes and pregnancy loss result in a lower than expected frequency of unbalanced offspring.

### Reciprocal translocations

Reciprocal translocation involves interchromosomal exchange. Either arm of any chromosome can be involved and the carriers are usually healthy. The medical significance is therefore usually for *future* generations, as carriers can produce chromosomally unbalanced fetuses.

### Insertional translocations

Insertional translocation involves insertion of a deleted segment interstitially at another location. It is extremely rare and balanced carriers are usually healthy, but may produce chromosomally unbalanced offspring with either a duplication or a deletion.

## Deletions

Deletion of part of a chromosome can be **interstitial** or **terminal**. Deletions can arise from two breaks, followed by faulty repair, from unequal crossing-over in a previous meiosis, or as a consequence of a translocation in a parent.

The smallest deletions detectable by **high-resolution banding** (see Chapter 43) are of about 3000 Kb (i.e. 3 million base pairs) and are generally characterized by mental handicap and multiple congenital malformations.

Several syndromes are ascribed to microscopically invisible **microdeletions** (see Chapter 35). When several genes are deleted together the term **contiguous gene syndrome** is applied.

## Ring chromosomes

If two breaks occur in the same chromosome the broken ends can fuse as a ring. Acentric rings are lost, but if the ring contains a centromere it can survive subsequent cell division. Clinically a ring represents two deletions. They can double by sister chromatid exchange, leading to effective trisomy, or be lost, resulting in monosomy.

## Duplications

Duplication is the presence of two adjacent copies of a chromosomal segment and can be either '**direct**', or '**inverted**'. Duplications may originate by unequal crossing-over in a previous meiosis, or as a consequence of translocation, inversion or presence of an iso-chromosome (see below) in a parent. Duplications are more common, but generally less harmful than deletions.

## Inversions

Inversions arise from two chromosomal breaks with end-to-end switching of the intervening segment. If this includes the centromere it is **pericentric**; if not, the inversion is **paracentric**. The medical significance of inversions lies in their capacity to lead to chromosomally unbalanced gametes following crossing-over.

## Isochromosomes

An isochromosome has a deletion of one chromosome arm, with duplication of the other. In live births the commonest involves the long arm of the X, resulting in Turner syndrome due to short arm monosomy (despite long arm trisomy). Most isochromosomes cause spontaneous abortion.

## Examples of deletions
### Prader–Willi and Angelman syndromes

The combined incidence of **Prader–Willi** and **Angelman syndromes** is 1/25 000 live births. Around 70% of patients have a deletion in the long arm of chromosome 15; in Prader–Willi this is in the paternal copy, in Angelman the maternal (see Chapter 19).

### Cri-du-chat syndrome

**Cri-du-chat syndrome** is so called because the malformed larynxes of these babies cause them to cry with a sound like a cat. They have profound learning disability, **hypertelorism** (widely spaced eyes), epicanthal folds, **strabismus**, low-set ears, low birth weight and failure to thrive. The cause is terminal deletion of the short arm of Chromosome 5 and it occurs in about 1/50 000 births.

### Wolf–Hirschhorn syndrome

**Wolf–Hirschhorn syndrome** also occurs in about 1/50 000 births, also with profound cognitive impairment, hypertelorism, epicanthal folds and low-set ears. Patients typically have a broad and prominent nose, cleft lip and palate, microcephaly, heart defects, convulsions and **hypospadias** (non-closure of the penile urethra). It is caused by terminal deletion of the short arm of Chromosome 4.

## Examples of translocations
### Down syndrome

About 4% of cases of Down syndrome are due to Robertsonian translocation between the long arms of Chromosome 21 and any other acrocentric, usually 14. In some cases one parent has a balanced version of the same translocation (see figure).

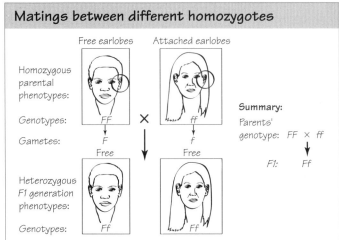

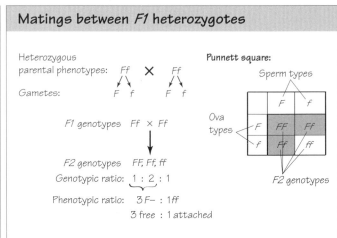

## Overview

Gregor Mendel's laws of inheritance were derived from experiments with plants, but they form the cornerstone of the whole science of genetics. Previously heredity was considered in terms of the transmission and mixing of 'essences', as suggested by Hippocrates over 2000 years before. But, unlike fluid essences that should blend in the offspring in all proportions, Mendel showed that the instructions for contrasting characters segregate and recombine in simple mathematical proportions. He therefore suggested that the hereditary factors are particulate.

Mendel postulated four new principles concerning **unit inheritance**, **dominance**, **segregation** and **independent assortment** that apply to most genes of all diploid organisms.

## The principle of unit inheritance

*Hereditary characters are determined by indivisible units of information (which we now call genes). An allele is one version of a gene.*

## The principle of dominance

*Alleles occur in pairs in each individual, but the effects of one allele may be masked by those of a dominant partner allele.*

## The principle of segregation

*During formation of the gametes the members of each pair of alleles separate, so that each gamete carries only one allele of each pair. Allele pairs are restored at fertilization.*

## Example

The earlobes of some people have an elongated attachment to the neck while others are free, a distinction determined by two alleles of the same gene, *f* for **attached**, *F* for **free**.

Consider a man carrying two copies of *F* (i.e. *FF*), with free earlobes, married to a woman with attached earlobes and two copies of *f* (i.e. *ff*). Both can produce only one kind of gamete, *F* for the man, *f* for the woman. All their children will have one copy of each allele, i.e. are *Ff*, and it is found that all such children have free earlobes because *F* is dominant to *f*. The children constitute the **first filial generation** or **F1 generation** (irrespective of the symbol for the gene under consideration). Individuals with identical alleles are **homozygotes**; those with different alleles are **heterozygotes**.

The **second filial**, or **F2, generation** is composed of the grandchildren of the original couple, resulting from mating of their offspring with partners of similar genotype. In each case both parents are heterozygotes, so both produce *F* and *f* gametes in equal numbers. This creates three genotypes in the F2: *FF*, *Ff* (identical to *fF*) and *ff*, **in the ratio: 1:2:1.**

Due to the dominance of *F* over *f*, dominant homozygotes are *phenotypically* the same as heterozygotes, so there are three offspring with free earlobes to each one with attached. ***The phenotypic ratio 3:1 is characteristic of the offspring of two heterozygotes.***

## The principle of independent assortment

*Different genes control different phenotypic characters and the alleles of different genes reassort independently of one another.*

## Example

Auburn and 'red' hair occur naturally only in individuals who are homozygous for a recessive allele *r*. Non-red is dominant, with the symbol *R*. All red-haired people are therefore *rr*, while non-red are either *RR* or *Rr*.

Consider the mating between an individual with red hair and attached earlobes (*rrff*) and a partner who is heterozygous at both genetic loci (*RrFf*). The recessive homozygote can produce only one kind of gamete, of genotype *rf*, but the double heterozygote can produce gametes of four genotypes: *RF*, *Rf*, *rF* and *rf*. Offspring of four genotypes are produced: *RrFf*, *Rrff*, *rrFf* and *rrff* and ***these are in the ratio 1:1:1:1.***

## Mating of a double heterozygote with a double recessive homozygote

Red hair is a homozygous recessive condition (*rr*).
Non-red is caused by *RR* or *Rr*.

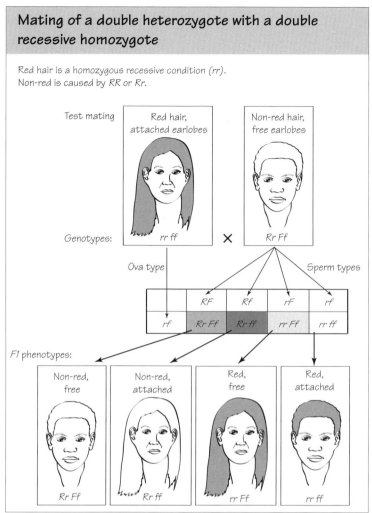

## Mating of a double heterozygote with a double dominant homozygote

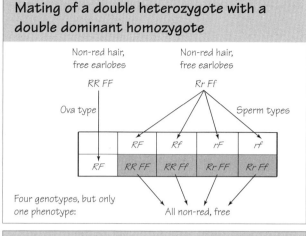

Four genotypes, but only one phenotype: All non-red, free

## Matings between double heterozygotes

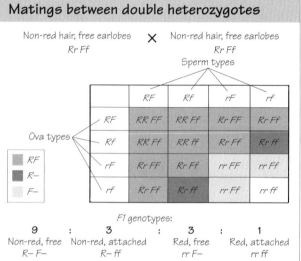

F1 genotypes:

| 9 | : | 3 | : | 3 | : | 1 |
|---|---|---|---|---|---|---|
| Non-red, free | | Non-red, attached | | Red, free | | Red, attached |
| R– F– | | R– ff | | rr F– | | rr ff |

---

These offspring also have phenotypes that are all different: non-red with free earlobes, non-red with attached, red with free, and red with attached, respectively.

### The test-mating

The mating described above, in which one partner is a double recessive homozygote (*rrff*), constitutes a **test-mating**, as his or her recessive alleles allow expression of all the alleles of the partner.

The value of such a test is revealed by comparison with matings in which the recessive partner is replaced by a double dominant homozygote (*RRFF*). The new partner can produce only one kind of gamete, of genotype *RF*, and four genotypically different offspring are produced, again in equal proportions: *RRFF, RRFf, RrFF* and *RrFf*. However, due to dominance all have non-red hair and free earlobes, so the genotype of the heterozygous parent remains obscure.

### Matings between double heterozygotes

The triumphant mathematical proof of Mendel laws was provided by matings between pairs of double heterozygotes. Each can produce four kinds of gametes: *RF, Rf, rF* and *rf*, which combined at random produce nine different genotypic combinations. ***Due to dominance there are four phenotypes, in the ratio 9 : 3 : 3 : 1 (total = 16)***. This allows us to predict the odds of producing:

1 a child with non-red hair and free earlobes (*R-F-*), as 9/16;
2 a child with non-red hair and attached earlobes (*R-ff*), as 3/16;
3 a child with red hair and free earlobes (*rrF-*), as 3/16; and
4 a child with red hair and attached earlobes (*rrff*), as 1/16.

### Biological support for Mendel's laws

The behaviour of Mendel's factors (alleles) coincides with the observed properties and behaviour of the chromosomes: (i) both occur in homologous pairs; (ii) at meiosis both separate, but reunite at fertilization; and (iii) the homologues of both segregate and recombine independently of one another. This coincidence is because the genes are components of the chromosomes.

### Exceptions to Mendel's laws

1 Sex-related effects (see Chapter 20).
2 Mitochondrial inheritance (see Chapter 20).
3 Genetic linkage (see Chapter 27).
4 Polygenic conditions (see Chapters 22, 23).
5 Incomplete penetrance (see Chapter 19).
6 Genomic imprinting (see Chapter 19).
7 Dynamic mutations (see Chapter 19).

# 17 Autosomal dominant inheritance

## Part of original pedigree for brachydactyly

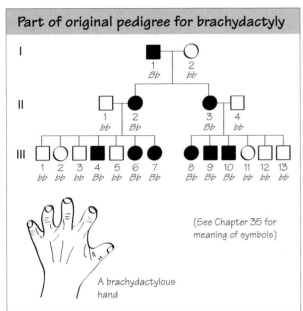

(See Chapter 35 for meaning of symbols)

A brachydactylous hand

## Achondroplasia

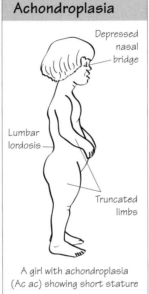

Depressed nasal bridge

Lumbar lordosis

Truncated limbs

A girl with achondroplasia (Ac ac) showing short stature

## Risk of transmission of achondroplasia in a marriage between two achondroplasics

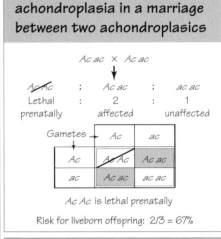

$$Ac\,ac \times Ac\,ac$$

| Ac Ac | ; | Ac ac | ; | ac ac |
|---|---|---|---|---|
| Lethal prenatally | : | 2 affected | : | 1 unaffected |

| Gametes ↓ | Ac | ac |
|---|---|---|
| Ac | Ac Ac | Ac ac |
| ac | Ac ac | ac ac |

Ac Ac is lethal prenatally

Risk for liveborn offspring: 2/3 = 67%

## Marfan syndrome

Adult heterozygote showing tall stature

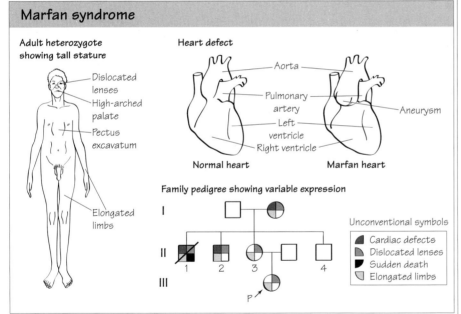

- Dislocated lenses
- High-arched palate
- Pectus excavatum
- Elongated limbs

### Heart defect

- Aorta
- Pulmonary artery
- Left ventricle
- Right ventricle
- Aneurysm

Normal heart       Marfan heart

### Family pedigree showing variable expression

Unconventional symbols
- ◣ Cardiac defects
- ◪ Dislocated lenses
- ◼ Sudden death
- ◺ Elongated limbs

P ↗

## Estimation of risk for offspring, autosomal dominant inheritance

Heterozygote paired with a normal homozygote (Bb × bb)

| Gametes ↓ | B | b |
|---|---|---|
| b | Bb | bb |
| b | Bb | bb |

Risk of B–: 2/4 = 50%

Heterozygote paired with another heterozygote (Bb × Bb)

| Gametes ↓ | B | b |
|---|---|---|
| B | BB | Bb |
| b | Bb | bb |

Risk of B–: 3/4 = 75%

Dominant homozygote paired with a normal homozygote (BB × bb)

| Gametes ↓ | B | B |
|---|---|---|
| b | Bb | Bb |
| b | Bb | Bb |

Risk of B–: 4/4 = 100%

## Overview

The best way to represent the distribution of affected individuals within a family is with a **pedigree diagram** (see Chapter 35). From this the mode of inheritance can often be easily deduced.

## The pedigree diagram

Females are symbolized by circles (○), males by squares (□), persons of unknown sex by diamonds (◇). Individuals affected by the disorder are represented by solid symbols (●, ■), those unaffected, by open symbols (○, □). Marriages or matings are indicated by horizontal lines linking male and female symbols. Offspring are shown beneath the parental symbols, in order of birth from left to right, linked to the mating line by a vertical, and numbered (1, 2, 3, etc.) from left to right in Arabic numerals. The generations are indicated in Roman numerals (I, II, III, etc.) from top to bottom on the left, with the earliest generation labelled I.

The patient who stimulated the investigation, the **propositus** (female: **proposita**), **proband**, or **index case**, is shown by an arrow (↗) with the letter P. The individual who sought genetic advice (the **consultand**) is shown by an arrow without the P. (N.B. in older texts the proband is indicated by an arrow alone). A diagonal line through the symbol indicates death.

## Rules for autosomal dominant inheritance
The following are the rules for simple **autosomal dominant inheritance**.
1 *Both males and females express the allele and can transmit it equally to sons and daughters.*
2 Excluding new mutations and non-penetrance (see Chapter 19), *every affected person has an affected parent* ('vertical' pattern of expression in the pedigree). *Direct transmission through three generations is practically diagnostic of a dominant.*
3 *In affected families, the ratio of affected to unaffected children is almost always 1:1.*
4 *If both parents are unaffected, all the children are unaffected.*

## Example
The first condition in humans for which the mode of inheritance was elucidated was **brachydactyly**, characterized by abnormally short phalanges (distal joints of fingers and toes).

In Mendelian symbols, the dominant allele *B* causes brachydactyly and every affected individual is either a homozygote (*BB*), or a heterozygote (*Bb*). In practice most are heterozygotes, because *brachydactyly is a rare trait* (i.e. <1/5000 births), *as are almost all dominant disease alleles.* Unrelated marriage partners are therefore usually recessive homozygotes (*bb*) and the mating can be represented:

*Bb*×*bb*
↓
*Bb, bb*
1:1

Dominant disease alleles are kept at low frequency since their carriers are less fit than normal homozygotes.

Matings between heterozygotes are the only kind that can produce homozygous offspring:

*Bb*×*Bb*
↓
***BB**, Bb, bb*
1:2:1, i.e. 3 affected: 1 unaffected.

*Dominant disease allele homozygotes are rare and with many disease alleles homozygosity is lethal*. Matings between heterozygotes may involve inbreeding (see Chapter 18), or occur when patients have met as a consequence of their disability (e.g. at a clinic for the disorder).
*All offspring of affected homozygotes are affected:*

*BB*×*bb*
↓
*Bb*

Unaffected members of affected families are normal homozygotes and so do not transmit the condition: *bb*×*bb* → *bb*

## Estimation of risk
In simply inherited autosomal dominant conditions where the diagnosis is secure, estimation of risk for the offspring of a family member can be based simply on the predictions of Mendel's laws. For example:
1 For the offspring of a heterozygote and a normal homozygote (*Bb*× *bb* → 1*Bb*; 1*bb*);
risk of *B*-= 1/2, or 50%.
2 For the offspring of two heterozygotes (*Bb*×*Bb* → 1*BB*; 2*Bb*; 1*bb*);
risk of *B*-= 3/4, or 75%.
3 For the offspring of a dominant homozygote with a normal partner (*BB*×*bb* → (*Bb*);
risk of *B*-= 1, or 100%.
Calculations involving dominant conditions can, however, be problematical as we usually do not know whether an affected offspring is homozygous or heterozygous (see Chapter 36).

## Clinical examples
Over 4000 autosomal dominant diseases are known, although few are common (>1/5000; see also Chapter 35).

### Achondroplasia (achondroplastic dwarfism)
**Achondroplasia** causes severe shortening of the long bones of the limbs, depression of the bridge of the nose and lumbar **lordosis** (exaggerated forward curvature of the spine). It is due to mutations in **fibroblast growth factor receptor**, **FGFR 3**, and is lethal prenatally in homozygotes. Liveborn offspring of two persons with achondroplasia (*Ac ac*) therefore have a two-thirds risk of being affected, not three-quarters (see figure).

### Acute intermittent porphyria
The porphyrias are characterized by occasional excretion of red porphyrin in the urine. Much of the time they are asymptomatic, but severe neurological symptoms can occur during starvation, or following consumption of certain chemicals. It is therefore an example of a **pharmacogenetic trait** (see Chapter 19).

### Marfan syndrome
Patients are tall, with long, thin limbs and fingers and dislocated eye lenses, **pectus excavatum** (funnel chest) and a high-arched palate. The aorta is susceptible to **aneurysm** (swelling) which if left untreated may lead to rupture. The underlying defect is in the protein **fibrillin-1**, in the periosteum, and connective tissue. Expression is variable and only some features may occur in any patient (see figure).

## Estimation of mutation rate
The frequency of dominant diseases in families with no prior cases can be used to estimate the natural frequency of new point mutations (see Chapter 29). This varies widely between genes, but averages about one event in any specific gene per 500 000 zygotes. Almost all point mutations arise in sperm, each containing around 40 000 genes (see Chapter 4). There are therefore about 40 000 mutations per 500 000 sperm and we can expect around 8% of viable sperm (and babies) to carry a new genetic mutation. However, only a minority of these occurs within genes that produce clinically significant effects, or would behave as dominant traits.

# 18 Autosomal recessive inheritance

### First-cousin marriage between heterozygotes

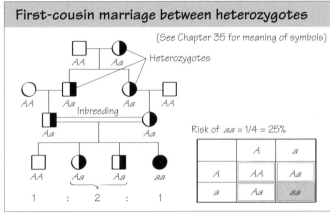

(See Chapter 35 for meaning of symbols)

Risk of *aa* = 1/4 = 25%

|  | *A* | *a* |
|---|---|---|
| *A* | *AA* | *Aa* |
| *a* | *Aa* | *aa* |

### Degrees of relationship with proband

Unconventional symbols:

◆ 1st degree: parents, offspring, siblings; 50% in common with proband

◇ 2nd degree: grandparents, grandchildren aunts, uncles, nephews, nieces; 25% in common with proband

◇ Third degree: first cousins: 12.5% in common with proband

(Marriage partners not all included)

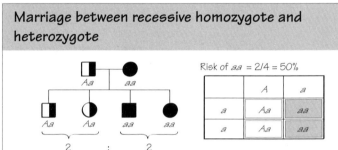

### Marriage between recessive homozygotes

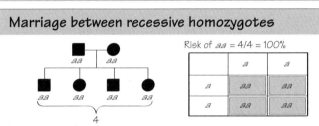

Risk of *aa* = 4/4 = 100%

|  | *a* | *a* |
|---|---|---|
| *a* | *aa* | *aa* |
| *a* | *aa* | *aa* |

### Marriage between recessive homozygote and heterozygote

Risk of *aa* = 2/4 = 50%

|  | *A* | *a* |
|---|---|---|
| *a* | *Aa* | *aa* |
| *a* | *Aa* | *aa* |

### Cumulative postnatal mortalities among 3442 offspring of first cousins and 5224 offspring of unrelated parents

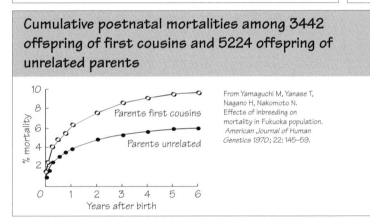

From Yamaguchi M, Yanase T, Nagano H, Nakomoto N. Effects of inbreeding on mortality in Fukuoka population. *American Journal of Human Genetics* 1970; 22: 145–59.

### A family pedigree showing two kinds of recessive deafness

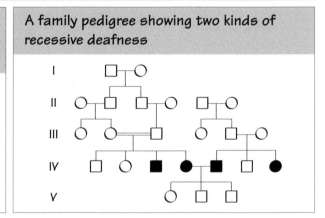

## Overview

The pedigree diagram for a family in which autosomal recessive disease is present differs markedly from those with other forms of inheritance. Recessive diseases can be relatively common, as heterozygous carriers can preserve and transmit disease alleles without adverse selection.

## Rules of autosomal recessive inheritance

The following are the rules for simple **autosomal recessive inheritance**:

1 *Both males and females are affected.*
2 *There are breaks in the pedigree* and typically *the pattern of expression is 'horizontal'* (i.e. sibs are affected, but parents are not).
3 *Affected children can be born to normal parents*, usually in the ratio of one affected to three unaffected.

4 *When both parents are affected all the children are affected.*
5 *Affected individuals with normal partners usually have only normal children.*

## Example

Homozygotes for oculocutaneous **albinism** (**albinos**) represent around 1 in 10 000 births. They have very pale hair and skin, blue or pink irides and red pupils. They suffer from **photophobia** (avoidance of light) and involuntary eye movements called **nystagmus**, related to faults in the neural connections between eye and brain. Their biochemical defect is in the enzyme **tyrosinase**, which normally converts tyrosine, through dihydroxy-phenylalanine (DOPA), into DOPA quinone, a precursor of the dark pigment, **melanin** (see Chapter 39).

Every albino is a recessive homozygote (**aa**) and most are born to phenotypically normal parents, who can also produce normal homozygotes and heterozygotes in the ratio of one dominant homozygote to two pigmented heterozygotes to one albino:

$Aa \times Aa \rightarrow 1AA : 2Aa : 1aa$; three pigmented : one albino

Matings between albinos produce only albino babies:

$aa \times aa \rightarrow aa$

Albinos with normally pigmented partners usually produce only pigmented offspring as the albinism allele is relatively rare:

$aa \times AA \rightarrow Aa$

Occasionally, however, a normally pigmented partner is a heterozygote and a half of the children of such matings are recessive homozygotes:

$aa \times Aa \rightarrow Aa, aa$; 1 pigmented : 1 albino

Superficially the latter pattern resembles that due to dominant heterozygotes with normal partners (see Chapter 17) and so is referred to as 'pseudodominance'.

Recessive diseases can be common in reproductively closed populations and molecular tests are used to identify unaffected carriers. The frequency of heterozygotes can be calculated from that of homozygotes by the **Hardy–Weinberg law** (see Chapter 26).

## Estimation of risk

Recessive homozygotes are produced by three kinds of mating, although the first of these is by far the most common.

1 **Two heterozygotes:** $Aa \times Aa \rightarrow 1AA : 2Aa : 1aa$; risk = 1/4, 0.25 or 25%.
2 **Recessive homozygote and heterozygote:** $aa \times Aa \rightarrow 1Aa : 1aa$; risk = 1/2, 0.5 or 50%.
3 **Two recessive homozygotes:** $aa \times aa \rightarrow aa$; risk = 1 or 100%.

## Clinical examples (see also Chapter 35)

### Cystic fibrosis
Cystic fibrosis is the most common recessive disease in Europeans, affecting one in 1800–2500 live births. It affects many systems of the body, but especially the lungs and pancreas and is lethal if untreated. The basic defect is in chloride ion transport.

### Tay–Sachs disease
The incidence of Tay–Sachs disease in American non-Jews is one in 360 000, but it is a hundred times as common (1 in 3600) in American Ashkenazi Jews. It affects the entire nervous system and is lethal, usually by the age of 2 years. The basic defect is a deficiency in **hexosaminidase A** (see Chapter 39).

### Spinal muscular atrophy
Spinal muscular atrophy is a progressive muscular weakness due to degeneration of the **anterior horn cells** of the spinal cord. The infantile form has a carrier frequency of 1/30 and is lethal by the age of 3 years. Juvenile forms are less common and progress more slowly. The collective incidence is 1/10 000 births.

### Phenylketonuria
In phenylketonuria, levels of phenylalanine and its breakdown products are elevated in the urine and blood, causing severe mental handicap, muscular hypertonicity and reduced pigmentation. The most usual defect is in **phenylalanine hydroxylase**, which normally converts dietary phenylalanine into tyrosine. Screening is routinely carried out at birth and homozygotes are given phenylalanine-free diets (see Chapter 42).

### Congenital deafness
There are many (>30) non-syndromic, autosomal recessive forms of congenital deafness that mimic one another at the gross phenotypic level in that all homozygotes are deaf. The frequency of heterozygotes is about 10%. *The children of two deaf parents may have perfect hearing if the parents are homozygous for mutant recessive alleles at different loci.*

If alleles $d$ and $e$ both cause deafness in the homozygous state, a mating between two deaf homozygotes could be represented:

$$\mathbf{dd}EE \quad \times \quad DD\mathbf{ee}$$
$$\text{deaf} \qquad\qquad \text{deaf}$$
$$\downarrow$$
$$DdEe$$

all offspring have normal hearing.

## Consanguineous matings

**Consanguinity** means that partners share at least one ancestor. **Inbreeding** between consanguineous partners is potentially harmful as it brings recessive alleles 'identical by descent' into the homozygous state in the offspring. **Incestuous** matings, e.g. between parent and child, or sibs (brother and sister) involve the greatest risk. The probability that a particular allele present in one individual is present also in an incestuous partner is 0.5. If each of us is heterozygous for one harmful (but non-lethal) recessive allele, the probability of a homozygous recessive offspring resulting from incestuous mating is:

$0.5 \times 0.25 = 0.125$, or 1/8.

For marriages between first cousins, the equivalent figures are 1/8 that an allele is shared and 1/32 (3%) that a homozygous baby will be produced. This accords with the observed frequency of recessive disease among offspring of first-cousin marriages, although that figure excludes early miscarriages.

Recessive disease occurs in outbred marriages at one-quarter of the square of the heterozygote frequency (see Chapter 26) and averages about 2% overall. In general, the rarer the disease and the greater the frequency of consanguineous marriages, the higher the proportion of recessive homozygotes produced by them.

The offspring of first-cousin marriages have 2.5 times as many congenital malformations and 70% higher postnatal mortality than those of outbred matings, both features of decreased vigour, known as **inbreeding depression**.

# 19 Intermediate inheritance

## Dominance and codominance in the ABO blood groups

| Genotypes | Description | Antigens on red cells | Blood groups |
|---|---|---|---|
| I^A^I^A | Homozygosity | A | A |
| I^A^I^0 | Dominance | A | A |
| I^B^I^B | Homozygosity | B | B |
| I^B^I^0 | Dominance | B | B |
| I^0^I^0 | Homozygosity | None | O |
| I^A^I^B | Codominance | A+B | AB |

## Age of onset of Huntington disease

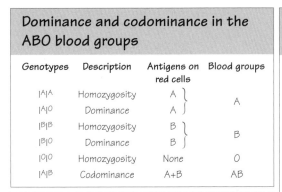

50% are affected by age 35 years

## A simplified pedigree for ectrodactyly, showing incomplete penetrance

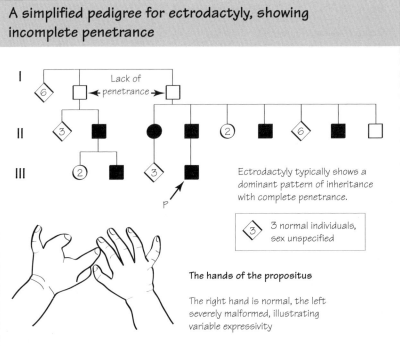

Ectrodactyly typically shows a dominant pattern of inheritance with complete penetrance.

◇3 — 3 normal individuals, sex unspecified

**The hands of the propositus**

The right hand is normal, the left severely malformed, illustrating variable expressivity

## Causation of Prader–Willi and Angelman syndromes

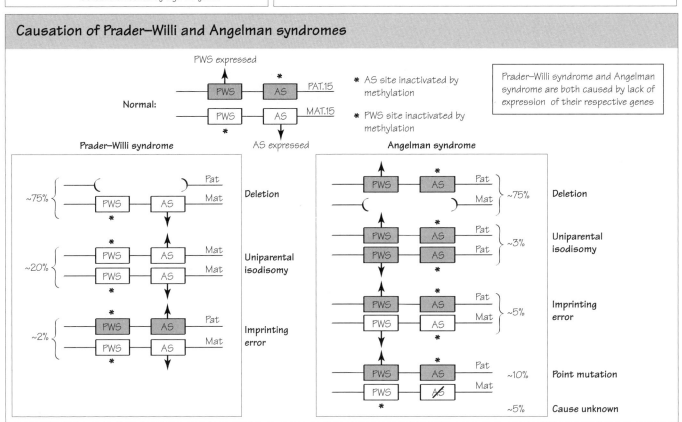

PWS expressed

Normal:
PWS  AS  PAT.15
PWS  AS  MAT.15

AS expressed

* AS site inactivated by methylation

* PWS site inactivated by methylation

Prader–Willi syndrome and Angelman syndrome are both caused by lack of expression of their respective genes

**Prader–Willi syndrome**

~75% — Deletion
~20% — Uniparental isodisomy
~2% — Imprinting error

**Angelman syndrome**

~75% — Deletion
~3% — Uniparental isodisomy
~5% — Imprinting error
~10% — Point mutation
~5% — Cause unknown

## Overview

**Incomplete dominance** refers to the situation when gene expression in heterozygotes is intermediate between that in the two homozygotes. In some cases neither of two alternative alleles is dominant, a situation called **codominance**. Alleles that are sometimes expressed and sometimes not, have **incomplete penetrance**, many alleles show **variable expressivity** and expression of some shows **delayed onset**. Some genes receive 'programming' during gametogenesis or development, called **genomic imprinting**.

## Dominance and codominance, the ABO blood groups

Dominance is defined in terms of which of two alternative alleles is expressed in the heterozygote.

In the ABO blood group system groups A, B, AB and O are distinguished by whether the red blood cells are agglutinated by anti-A or anti-B antibody (see Chapter 25). Group O cells have a precursor glycosphingolipid embedded in their surfaces which is elaborated differentially in A, B and AB by the products of alleles $I^A$ and $I^B$ (see Chapter 33).

The erythrocytes of both $I^B$ homozygotes and $I^B/I^O$ heterozygotes are agglutinated by anti-B antibody, so both are Group B. Similarly Group A includes both $I^A$ homozygotes and $I^A/I^O$ heterozygotes. Alleles $I^A$ and $I^B$ are both dominant to $I^O$.

The red cells of $I^O$ homozygotes are not agglutinated by antibodies directed against A or B. They belong to Group O.

The red cells of Group AB individuals carry both A and B antigens. They are agglutinated by *both* anti-A and anti-B, and are therefore Group AB. Since both are expressed together, alleles $I^A$ and $I^B$ are **codominant**.

The alleles of several other blood groups, the tissue antigens of the HLA system, the electrophoretic variants of many proteins and the DNA markers (see Part III) can also be considered codominant, as their properties are assessed directly, irrespective of expression.

## Incomplete dominance, sickle cell disease

Alpha- and beta-globin, together with haem and iron, make up the **haemoglobin** of our red blood cells. The normal allele for β-globin is called HbA and the **sickle cell allele**, HbS, differs from it by one base (see Chapter 30). In HbS homozygotes the abnormal haemoglobin aggregates, causing the red cells to collapse into the shape of a sickle and clog small blood vessels. **Sickle cell disease** is characterized by anaemia, intense pain, and vulnerability to infection.

Heterozygotes have both normal (A) and abnormal (S) haemoglobin molecules in their erythrocytes, which stay undistorted most of the time, allowing them to live a normal life. At this level HbA is dominant to HbS. However, under conditions of severe oxygen stress, a proportion do undergo sickling and this causes transient symptoms similar to those of homozygotes. On this basis HbS is classified as **incompletely dominant**.

Heterozygotes with the so-called **sickle cell trait** have a remarkable ability to tolerate *falciparum* malaria (see Chapter 25).

## Pleiotropy, expressivity and penetrance

**Pleiotropy** describes the expression of several different phenotypic features by a single allele. Most genes have pleiotropic alleles.

Patients with **Marfan syndrome** frequently do not show all its features and those that are shown can vary in severity (see Chapter 17). This is called **variable expressivity**.

Some apparently dominant alleles are not always expressed. **Ectrodactyly**, in which formation of the middle elements of hands and feet is variably disrupted, is caused by such a **dominant allele of reduced penetrance** (see figure).

**Degree of penetrance** is the percentage of carriers of a specific allele that show the relevant phenotype. For example, about 75% of women with certain mutations in the BRCA1 gene develop breast or ovarian cancer. The penetrance of those mutations therefore is 75%.

**Pharmacogenetic traits** are a special case of penetrance and expressivity in which the environmental agent that reveals the deficient allele is a drug (see Chapter 25).

## Genomic imprinting

**Imprinting** is a mechanism that ensures expression in an individual of either the maternal, or the paternal copy of a chromosomal region, but not both. It probably applies to only a small number of genes.

### Prader–Willi and Angelman syndromes

A microdeletion of Chromosome 15 causes Prader–Willi syndrome if in the paternal copy, but a distinctly different condition, Angelman syndrome, when that deletion is in the maternal copy. Prader–Willi syndrome patients show compulsive eating, obesity and mild to moderate neurodevelopmental delay; in Angelman syndrome, patients' neurodevelopmental delay is severe, they have uncoordinated movements and compulsive laughter.

This effect probably involves two adjacent genes that normally are differentially inactivated (by methylation) during the production of sperm and oocytes, respectively. In sperm the Angelman syndrome site (the gene for **ubiquitin protein ligase**) is inactivated, but the Prader–Willi syndrome site is not. In oocytes the Prader–Willi syndrome site is inactivated while the Angelman syndrome remains active. Normal development requires one active copy of each.

Occasionally embryos arise with **uniparental isodisomy** (see Chapter 14). If both copies of Chromosome 15 are paternal in origin, Angelman syndrome results. Similarly, Prader–Willi results when the Isodisomic 15 is maternal.

### Molar pregnancies

**Hydatidiform moles** are grossly abnormal embryonal tissue masses that can develop following simultaneous fertilization of one oocyte by two sperm. They can invade uterine muscle to cause **choriocarcinoma**. A 'complete mole' has two sets of paternal chromosomes only. 'Partial moles' are triploid.

### Mosaicism

**Mosaicism** refers to the existence in the body of more than one genetically distinct cell line following a single fertilization event (cf. **chimaerism**, in which different cell lines result from multiple fertilizations). Both mosaicism and chimaerism can produce incidence patterns that depart from the general rules.

### Delayed onset

**Huntington disease** can remain unexpressed until 30–50 years and is an example of a **disease of late onset**. Patients then undergo progressive degeneration of the nervous system, with uncontrolled movements and mental deterioration (see Chapter 30).

### Diagram of the X and Y chromosomes showing regions of homology and the map locations of some significant genes

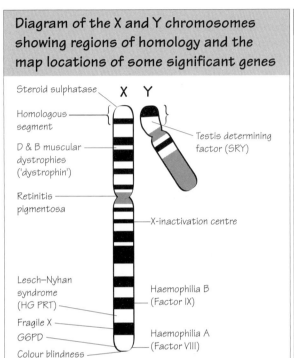

### X chromosome inactivation and somatic mosaicism

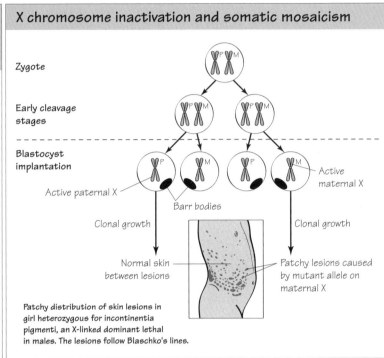

Patchy distribution of skin lesions in girl heterozygous for incontinentia pigmenti, an X-linked dominant lethal in males. The lesions follow Blaschko's lines.

### X-linked recessive inheritance

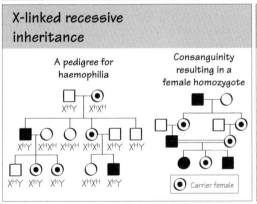

A pedigree for haemophilia

Consanguinity resulting in a female homozygote

⊙ Carrier female

### X-linked dominant inheritance

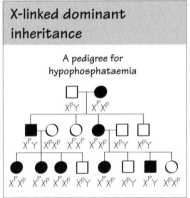

A pedigree for hypophosphataemia

### Mitochondrial inheritance

Theoretical pedigree for a family with MERRF, showing maternal inheritance and variable expression due to heteroplasmy

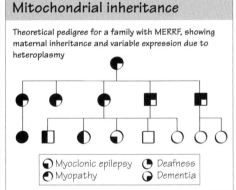

Myoclonic epilepsy — Deafness
Myopathy — Dementia

### Overview

Men and women differ in sex chromosome constitution, physiology and the gametes they produce. All three factors create features of inheritance that relate to sex, but most so-called 'sex-linked' disorders' are caused by X-linked recessives in males.

### X-linked recessive inheritance

**Rules**

1 *The incidence of disease is very much higher in males than females.*
2 *The mutant allele is passed from an affected man to all of his daughters, but they do not express it.*
3 *A heterozygous 'carrier' woman passes the allele to half of her sons, who express it, and half of her daughters who do not.*
4 *The mutant allele is never passed from father to son.*

**Example: Haemophilia A (classic haemophilia)** causes failure of blood clotting due to deficiency in **antihaemophilic globulin** or **blood clotting Factor VIII**.

A single copy of the normal allele is adequate for function, so the mutation is recessive and heterozygous females are normal. Males being **hemizygous** are affected, the incidence being about 1/10 000 male births.

Female homozygotes occur in the general population at a frequency equal to the square of that of affected males, i.e. 1/100 million. In inbreeding situations or when partners meet as a consequence of the mutant allele, they are found at higher frequency.

A man receives his Y chromosome from his father and passes a copy to every son. He receives his X from his mother and passes a copy to every daughter. Both mother and daughter are therefore **obligate**

**carriers** of any X-linked recessive expressed by the man. This pattern is sometimes referred to as **criss-cross inheritance**.

## Estimation of risk for offspring

### 1 Haemophiliac man and normal woman

$X^h Y \times X^H X^H \rightarrow$ normal sons ($X^H Y$) and carrier daughters ($X^H X^h$), ratio 1:1.

There is no risk of haemophilia in the children.

### 2 Carrier woman and normal man

$X^H X^h \times X^H Y \rightarrow$ normal daughters ($X^H X^H$), carrier daughters ($X^H X^h$), normal sons ($X^H Y$) and affected sons ($X^h Y$), in the ratio 1:1:1:1.

The risk of haemophilia in the offspring is 1/4.

### 3 Haemophiliac man and carrier woman

$X^h Y \times X^H X^h \rightarrow$ carrier daughters ($X^H X^h$), affected daughters ($X^h X^h$), normal sons ($X^H Y$) and affected sons ($X^h Y$), in the ratio 1:1:1:1.

The overall risk is 2/4 or 1/2.

### 4 Haemophiliac woman and normal man

$X^h X^h \times X^H Y \rightarrow$ Carrier daughters ($X^H X^h$) and affected sons ($X^h Y$), in the ratio 1:1.

All the sons are affected, and all the daughters are carriers; the risk is 1/2.

## Other examples (see also Chapter 35)

*Red blindness and green blindness*
These conditions are caused by highly homologous genes in tandem array on the X chromosome. About 8% of British men and 0.6% of British women are affected.

*Becker and Duchenne muscular dystrophies*
These involve different mutations of the **dystrophin** gene. **Duchenne** is the more severe and is usually lethal in adolescence. It is indicated by the **Gower sign** when a child climbs up his or her own body when standing from the prone position, because strength is retained longer in the upper than the lower limbs.

*Fragile X syndrome*
This is one of most important causes of severe learning difficulties in boys. In cell cultures the X chromosome tends to break at the mutant site.

*G6PD deficiency*
The frequency of this deficiency varies enormously between populations due to past selection for resistance to malaria (see Chapter 25).

## X-linked dominant disorders

X-linked dominant disorders are all rare.

### Rules

1 *The condition is expressed and transmitted by both sexes.*
2 *The condition occurs twice as frequently in females as in males.*
3 *An affected man passes the condition to every daughter, but never to a son.*
4 *An affected woman passes the condition to every son and half her daughters.*

**Example: Hypophosphataemia** or **vitamin D-resistant rickets** (see also Chapter 35).

## Y-linked or Holandric inheritance

DNA sequencing indicates at least 20 genes on the Y chromosome, several concerned with male sexual function. There are no known Y-linked diseases.

**Rule:** *Genes on the Y chromosome are expressed in and transmitted only by males, to all their sons.*

**Example:** The **testis determining factor or SRY gene** (see Chapter 2); the **H–Y tissue antigen**.

## Pseudoautosomal inheritance

**Rule:** *Genes on the homologous segments of the X and Y are transmitted by women equally to both sexes, but by a man predominantly to offspring of one sex.*

**Example: Steroid sulphatase deficient X-linked ichthyosis** (scaly skin).

## Sex limitation and sex influence

Some alleles are carried on the autosomes, but are limited or influenced by sex physiologically or for anatomical reasons (Table 20.3).

## Mitochondrial inheritance

Mitochondrial inheritance reflects the fact that a zygote receives all its functional mitochondria from the oocyte.

### Rules

1 *Typically the condition is passed from a mother to all her children.*
2 *The condition is never transmitted by men.*

Symptoms *can* vary between mother and offspring, and between sibs, due to **heteroplasmy**, i.e. variable representation of different mitochondrial populations.

### Example

A form of progressive blindness called **Leber hereditary optic neuropathy** (**LHON**); **MELAS**: mitochondrial myopathy, encephalopathy, lactic acidosis and stroke-like episodes; **MERRF**: myoclonic epilepsy with ragged red fibres; **KSS**: Kearns–Sayre syndrome.

## X chromosome inactivation

X chromosome inactivation (see Chapter 12) can sometimes cause expression of X-linked recessive alleles in heterozygous women. Heterozygosity is revealed if she produces both normal and affected sons or displays patches of tissue expressing alternative alleles (see figure).

# 21 Congenital abnormalities

## Relative frequency of birth defects in girls and boys

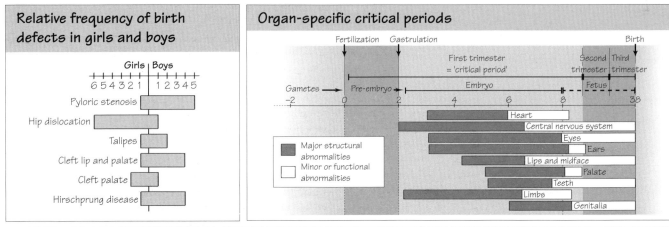

## Organ-specific critical periods

## Major birth defects (total 30–40/1000 births)

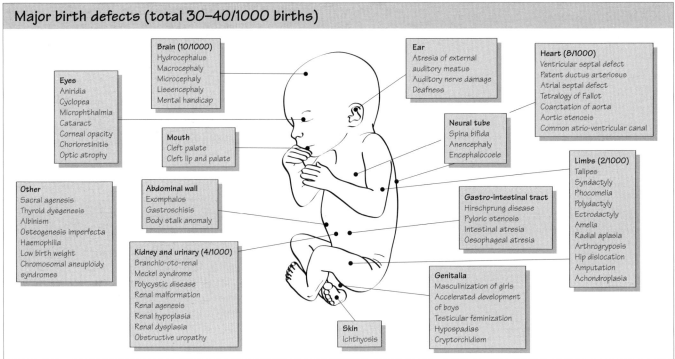

## Overview

The word '**congenital**' means 'existing at birth' and includes all 'birth defects' regardless of causation. Congenital abnormalities account for approximately 21% of all infant deaths and are a major contributor to later disability. The frequency of abnormalities is initially high, but most are lost by natural abortion. At birth 0.7% of babies have *multiple major* abnormalities, 2–3% a *single major* defect and 14% a *single minor* defect. Incidence of some abnormalities differs considerably between the sexes (see figure). Probably 15–25% of congenital abnormalities have a recognized genetic and 10% a recognized environmental basis, while in 20–25% the basis is multifactorial. Twinning accounts for 0.5–1.0% (see Chapter 24) and 40–60% are **idiopathic**, i.e.

of unknown causation. Extrinsic agents that cause birth defects are called **teratogens**.

## Principles of teratogenesis

1 Susceptibility to a teratogen depends on the genotype of the zygote.
2 Maternal genotype and health status affect the metabolism of drugs, resistance to infection and other metabolic processes.
3 Susceptibility depends on developmental stage at time of exposure.
4 Severity depends on dose and duration of exposure to teratogen.
5 Individual teratogens have specific modes of action.
6 Abnormality is expressed as malformation, growth retardation, functional disorder or death.

## Classification of defects

1 **Malformations** are due to errors occurring in the initial formation of structures.
2 **Disruptions** are due to destructive processes operating after an organ has formed.
3 **Deformations** are distortions due to abnormal mechanical forces.
4 **Dysplasias** are abnormalities in the organization of cells into tissues.
5 **Sequences** are cascades of effects originating from an earlier abnormality.
6 **Syndromes** are groups of anomalies that consistently occur together.

## Genotype of the zygote

Duplication or deficiency of even part of a chromosome may cause embryonic or fetal death, postnatal **neurodevelopmental delay**, pre- or postnatal **growth delay** and/or **dysmorphology** (see Chapter 37).

## Health status of the mother

The most important maternal predisposing conditions are **alcoholism, phenylketonuria, insulin dependent diabetes mellitus (IDDM)**, systemic **lupus erythematosis (SLE)** and **Graves disease.**

## Timing and aetiology

### Pre-embryo

Damage to the pre-embryo generally results in spontaneous abortion or regulative repair, so few errors in newborns are ascribable to preimplantation damage. The following are exceptions:
1 **Monozygotic twinning.**
2 **Germ layer defects**, e.g. **ectodermal dysplasias** affecting skin, nails, hair, teeth and stature.

### Embryo

The **first trimester** (i.e. the first 3 months) is **the critical period**, as it is characterized by many delicate and complex tissue interactions.

The following are particularly important:
1 **Failure of cell migration**, e.g. neural crest cells: **Waardenburg syndrome.**
2 **Failure of embryonic induction**, e.g. **anophthalmia** (absence of eyes).
3 **Failure of tube closure**, e.g. the neural tube remaining open in the lumbar region in **spina bifida** and anteriorly in **anencephaly.**
4 **Developmental arrest**, e.g. **cleft lip** (see Chapters 22 and 23).
5 **Failure of tissue fusion**, e.g. **cleft palate** (see Chapters 22 and 23).
6 **Defective morphogenetic fields**, e.g. **sirenomelia** (mermaid-like fusion of legs).
The foundations of **consequent disturbances** can be laid at this stage, e.g. the **Potter sequence** due to **oligohydramnios,** or deficiency of amniotic fluid caused by renal agenesis, polycystic kidney disease, urethral obstruction, or fluid leakage. A fetus growing in a fluid-deprived space may suffer compression, immobility, breech presentation, facial and limb deformities, growth deficiency and pulmonary hypoplasia.

### Fetus

During the fetal period the organ systems grow and mature towards a functional state and there is extensive **programmed cell death**, or **apoptosis**. Abnormalities are largely in growth, **ossification** of the skeleton and the ordering of neural connections. The latter is of particular importance as errors can cause mental dysfunction.

Causes include:
1 **Absence of normal apoptosis**, e.g. finger webbing.
2 **Disturbances in tissue resorption**, e.g. **anal atresia** (imperforate anus).
3 **Failure of organ movement**, e.g. **cryptorchism** (or **cryptorchidism**: failure of descent of the testes).
4 **Destruction of formed structures**, e.g. **phocomelia** (seal-like arms), due to interference in blood supply.
5 **Hypoplasia** (reduced proliferation), e.g. **achondroplasia**.
6 **Hyperplasia** (enhanced proliferation), e.g. **macrosomia (large body size)** due to maternal diabetes mellitus.
7 **Constriction** by **amniotic bands** (strands of broken amnion), e.g. limb amputation.
8 **Restriction of movement**, e.g. **talipes** (club foot).

## Medicines

Teratogenic medicines include:
1 **Abortifacients** (agents intended to induce abortion), e.g. the folic acid antagonist **aminopterin.**
2 **Antiabortifacients**, e.g. **diethylstibestrol**: malformations of reproductive systems.
3 **Androgens** (male sex hormones): masculinization of external genitalia of girls.
4 **Anticonvulsants** used by epileptics: **trimethadone, diphenylhydantoin, valproate, phenytoin, carbamazepine.**
5 **Sedatives** and **tranquillizers: thalidomide, lithium.**
6 **Anticancer drugs: methotrexate, aminopterin.**
7 **Antibiotics: streptomycin** can cause inner ear deafness; **tetracycline** inhibits skeletal calcification.
8 **Anticoagulants: warfarin, dicumarol.**
9 **Antihypertensive agents: ACE inhibitors.**
10 **Antithyroid drugs.**
11 **Vitamin A analogues**, e.g. **retinoids** used to treat acne.

## Non-prescription drugs

**Alcohol** can cause 'fetal alcohol syndrome' with poor postnatal growth, mental retardation, heart defects and facial midline hypoplasia. **LSD (lysergic acid diethylamide), 'Angel dust' or PCP (phenylcyclidine), quinine** and birth control pills are all **teratogenic. Tobacco** smoking causes growth retardation and premature delivery.

## Environmental chemicals

Lead, methylmercury and **hypoxia** are the best recognized hazards.

## Infection

Some infections during pregnancy lead to fetal abnormality:
1 **Viruses**: *Rubella* (German measles), *Cytomegalovirus, Herpes simplex, Parvovirus, Varicella* (chicken pox).
2 **Protozoa**: *Toxoplasma gondii.*
3 **Bacteria**: *Treponema pallidum* (syphilis).

## Physical agents

These include: **hyperthermia** due to infection or hot baths. **Ionizing radiation** and **X-rays** can cause developmental errors secondary to genetic damage (see Chapter 29).

## Polygenic basis of stature

In this theoretical model height is considered to be controlled by two genes, each with two codominant alleles, A/a and B/b. Alleles A and B make positive, and a and b negative contributions to height. The basis of a normal distribution is created, with individuals of medium height most frequent

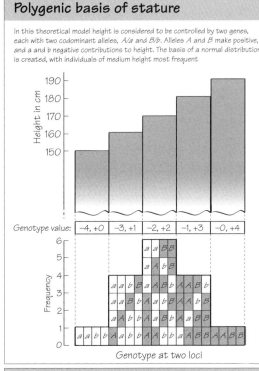

## Normal distribution of stature in men

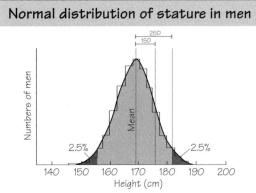

## The multifactorial threshold model

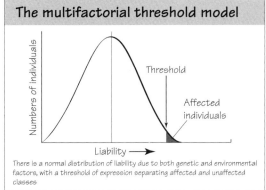

There is a normal distribution of liability due to both genetic and environmental factors, with a threshold of expression separating affected and unaffected classes

## Recurrence risks in relatives

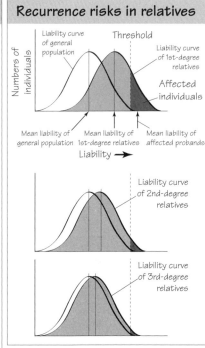

## The effect of sex-related differential thresholds on recurrence risks (based on pyloric stenosis)

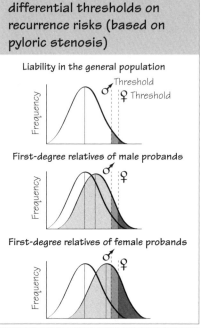

## Formation of the upper lip and palate

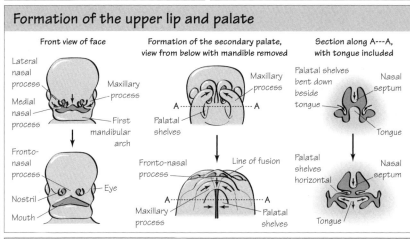

## The threshold model applied to creation of cleft palate

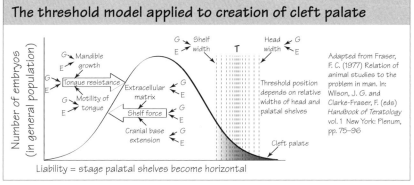

Liability = stage palatal shelves become horizontal

Adapted from Fraser, F. C. (1977) Relation of animal studies to the problem in man. In: Wilson, J. G. and Clarke-Fraser, F. (eds) Handbook of Teratology vol. 1 New York: Plenum, pp. 75–96

## Overview

Mendelian traits show **discontinuous variation** in that alternative phenotypes are distinctly different. With some characters variation is **continuous**, with no natural boundaries. This chapter explains how discontinuous and continuous variation can be seen as two aspects of the same genetic system.

## Continuous variation

Quantitative characters such as height, skin colour and intelligence quotient (IQ) typically show continuous variation, their frequency distributions approximating a **normal curve**. Such patterns are generated by the combined action of many genes, i.e. they are **polygenic** (see figure), or together with environmental factors, **multifactorial**.

Genetic experiments with other species show that quantitative variation at just a few loci can produce a **normal distribution** definable in terms of its **mean** and **standard deviation**. Individuals that exceed two standard deviations above or below the population mean (i.e. 2.5% at either extreme) are regarded clinically as 'abnormal'. The concept of a **normal range** is fundamental in paediatrics, where height, weight, head circumference, etc. are routinely measured in monitoring a child's development (see Chapter 37).

## Discontinuous variation: threshold traits

Sometimes too few individuals are affected for familial patterns to be interpreted. One explanation conceives an underlying normal distribution of **liability** to disease, due to an assemblage of harmful genetic and environmental factors and truncated by a threshold of disease manifestation. We all lie somewhere within each liability range, affected people to the right of the threshold, and all those near the threshold having a greater than average probability of producing diseased offspring. Such conditions are known as **multifactorial threshold traits**.

### Rules for identification of a multifactorial threshold trait

*1 Disorders can be common (>1/5000 births; although they can also be rare!)*. By comparison, seriously disabling, fully penetrant, dominant conditions are usually selected out by disease, reduced fertility, early death or failure to mate.

*2 The disorder runs in families, but there is no distinctive pattern of inheritance.*

*3 The concordance rate in monozygotic (MZ) twins is significantly greater than in dizygotic (DZ)* (see Chapter 24).

*4 The frequency of disease in second degree relatives is much lower than in first degree, but declines less rapidly for more distant relatives.* (See CL ± P below).

*5 Recurrence risk is proportional to the number of family members already affected.* This is because the occurrence of several affected family members indicates a particularly high concentration of harmful alleles.

*6 Recurrence risk is proportional to the severity of the condition in the proband.* This is because severity of expression and recurrence risk both depend on the concentration of adverse alleles (see CL ± P below).

*7 Recurrence risk is higher for relatives of the less susceptible sex.* This is because disease expression in the less susceptible sex requires the higher concentration of harmful alleles.

## Malformations

### Examples (see also Chapter 24)

*Cleft lip with or without cleft palate*

**Cleft lip with or without cleft palate** (CL ± P) is causally distinct from **cleft palate** (CP) alone. It is caused by failure of fusion of the frontal and maxillary processes and includes chromosomal, teratogenic, monogenic and multifactorial forms.

A critical feature is the maturity of the cells on the surfaces of the lateral and medial processes in relation to their relative physical locations. Fusion of lateral and medial elements requires unimpeded movement of the palatal shelves past the tongue.

CL ± P affects about 1/1000 Europeans (0.1%), twice as many Japanese and half as many Afro-Americans. Recurrence risks in relatives of different degree (see Chapter 18) are:
- first degree = 4%;
- second degree = 0.6%;
- third degree = 0.3% (Rule 4; see figure).

Severity of expression varies from unilateral cleft lip alone (UCL) to bilateral cleft lip with cleft palate (BCL+P). The incidence of CL ± P (of all types) in first degree relatives is directly related to severity of expression in the proband (Rule 6):
- proband has UCL, incidence is 4%;
- proband has UCL+P, incidence is 5%;
- proband has BCL, incidence is 7%;
- proband has BCL+P, incidence is 8%;
- 60–80% of patients are male and the incidence in sibs of male probands is 5.5%;
- 20–40% of patients are female and the incidence in their sibs is 7% (Rule 7).

*Pyloric stenosis*

Pyloric stenosis involves abnormal musculature in the pyloric sphincter, leading to feeding problems, with projectile vomiting.

It occurs in 5/1000 male, but only 1/1000 female infants. Affected females are three times as likely as males to have affected offspring (Rule 7). The sons of affected women have the highest risk, at about 20% (see figure).

*Spina bifida and anencephaly*

These occur due to failure of closure of the neural tube (see Chapter 11), which in genetically susceptible families relates to folic acid deficiency. In Northern England the natural incidence was about 1/200; it is now reduced to less than 1/1000 after vitamin supplementation and termination of affected pregnancies (see Chapters 40, 47 and 48).

*Cleft palate (CP)*

Cleft palate alone affects rather more girls than boys and accounts for 1/2000 malformed births.

*Congenital heart disease*

Ninety per cent of cases are multifactorial, affecting eight babies per 1000.

**The common disorders of adult life**

## Overview

Pedigree analysis is unhelpful with the commonest serious diseases because simple inheritance patterns are rarely found. The traditional explanation has been polygenic causation, i.e. that there are *many* causative genes, each of *minor* effect, all acting *together*. They are sometimes classed as multifactorial threshold traits (see Chapter 22), but with new knowledge such explanations are becoming progressively less convincing.

Some common diseases are **oligogenic**, i.e. there are *a few major genes acting together*. In most cases this is probably just two autosomal dominants (Table 23.1). In many others a *dominant allele of incomplete penetrance is acting alone*. They are also usually **genetically heterogeneous**, i.e. different genetic loci are important in different families.

## Methodolgy
### Twin studies

If a disease has a major genetic component, identical, or **MZ**, twin pairs tend to have a high degree of **concordance** for disease (i.e. both are usually affected), whereas in non-identical, **DZ**, twins concordance is much lower. The degree of MZ concordance indicates the penetrance of the genotype, while DZ concordance reveals the number of causative loci simultaneously involved (see Chapter 24). If MZ and DZ concordances are similar, genotype is unimportant.

### Family studies

If there is genetic causation the relative risk for family members is higher than in the general population and increases with closeness of relationship (Table 23.2; see Chapter 18).

### Adoption studies

Incidence of disease in children of affected parents adopted into unaffected families can show to what extent genetic predisposition is causative, as compared to home environment.

### Population studies

Study of migrant groups, or variant ethnic groups in the same environment can reveal genetic involvement.

### Polymorphism association analysis

This approach seeks association of disease with specific alleles of a **candidate gene** (see Chapter 28).

### Linkage studies

**Linkage** studies look for co-transmission of disease with polymorphisms of possible linked **genetic markers** (see Chapters 27 and 28).

### Biochemical studies

Biochemical studies investigate abnormal activity of enzymes involved in implicated biochemical pathways (Chapter 39).

### Animal models

Animal models provide biochemical insight and help in gene mapping by providing homologous chromosome segments as comparators.

## Examples
### Essential hypertension

High blood pressure with no obvious cause is called **essential hyper-**

**Table 23.1** Significant properties of some common diseases.*

| | Frequency/1000 | MZ conc. (%) | DZ conc. (%) | n | P |
|---|---|---|---|---|---|
| Coronary artery disease | Up to 500 | 46 | 12 | 1 or 2 | 0.6 |
| Atopic diathesis | 250 | 50 | 4 | 3 | 0.7 |
| Unipolar affective disorder | 20–250 | 54 | 19 | 1 | 0.7 |
| Essential hypertension | 100 | 30 | 10 | 1 | 0.5 |
| NIDDM | 30–70 | 100 | 10 | 2 | 1.0 |
| Rheumatoid arthritis | 20 | 30 | 5 | 2 | 0.5 |
| Epilepsy | 10 | 37 | 10 | 1 or 2 | 0.5 |
| Schizophrenia | 10 | 45 | 13.0 | 1 | 0.6 |
| Psoriasis | 10 | 61 | 13.0 | 1 or 2 | 0.75 |
| Bipolar affective disorder | 4 | 79 | 24 | 1 | 0.9 |
| IDDM | 2 | 30–40 | 6 | 2 | 0.5 |
| Multiple sclerosis | 1 | 20–30 | 6 | 2 | 0.4 |
| Leprosy | Varies | 60 | 20 | 1 | 0.75 |
| Tuberculosis | Varies | 87 | 26 | 1 | 0.9 |
| Measles | Varies | 97 | 94 | 0.0 | — |

Conc., concordance; NIDDM, non-insulin dependent diabetes mellitus; IDDM, insulin dependent diabetes mellitus; n, number of major genes acting in a monogenic or together in an oligogenic system, estimated from comparison of twin concordances (see Chapter 24). These data give no indication of genetic heterogeneity. P, approximate penetrance, estimated from MZ concordance (see Chapter 24).
*This table is intended to present only a general picture; actual frequencies and concordances vary in different published reports.

**tension**. This can lead to stroke (cerebral haemorrhage), renal and coronary artery disease. Up to 40% of 70-year-olds are hypertensive.

Twin concordance rates and increased risk in relatives suggest monogenic autosomal dominant inheritance in a few families. It frequently shows familial clusters, but other inheritance patterns are more complex. Biochemical studies implicate the **sodium–potassium transmembrane pump**, the **angiotensin I converting enzyme (ACE)** and the **angiotensin II type I receptor**. Mapping studies indicate three major susceptibility loci.

High sodium intake, obesity, alcohol and lack of exercise all contribute to the condition.

## Coronary artery disease

Coronary artery disease (CAD) accounts for up to 50% of deaths in economically developed countries. Lipid deposition in the coronary arteries causes fibrous conversion (**atherosclerosis**), failure of blood supply (**ischaemia**) and death of heart muscle (**myocardial infarction**).

Genetic involvement, with incomplete penetrance, is indicated by twin concordance rates and family studies. Fifteen per cent of cases show autosomal dominant inheritance and at least four loci are independently involved.

Predisposing conditions include **familial combined hyperlipidaemia (FCH)**, **familial hypercholesterolaemia (FH)** and point mutations in **apoB-100** (all inherited as autosomal dominants), **diabetes mellitus** and **hypertension** (see above).

Causative environmental factors include smoking, cholesterol intake and lack of exercise.

## Diabetes mellitus

**Diabetes mellitus** is characterized by **hyperglycaemia** (excess glucose in the blood) that can cause many health problems including coma and death.

**1 Insulin dependent diabetes mellitus (IDDM), Type 1**, or **juvenile onset diabetes** affects 3–7% of Western adults, the peak age of onset being 12 years. Twin concordance rates and familial patterns indicate a genetic basis. Two loci are especially important: **IDDM-1** and **IDDM-2**, that together account for 40–50% of genetic predisposition. These

concern autoimmune susceptibility (see Chapter 33) and insulin production.

**2 Non-insulin dependent diabetes mellitus (NIDDM)** or **Type 2 diabetes** is 10 times as common as IDDM, with an older age of onset. Twin concordance indicates a strong genetic basis and high penetrance. Linkage studies suggest three susceptibilty loci.

**3 Maturity onset diabetes of the young (MODY)** affects 1–2% of diabetics in early adulthood. Some families show autosomal dominant inheritance and six or more loci are indicated.

## Atopic diathesis

**Atopic diathesis** constitutes an exuberant IgE response to low levels of antigen (see Chapter 33). One in four of the population share an autosomal dominant allele that is possibly imprinted (see Chapter 17) as incidence is highest in the offspring of affected mothers. Patients develop 'hay fever', eczema and asthma.

## Schizophrenia

**Schizophrenia** is a seriously disabling psychosis affecting about 1% of the population. Twin concordance rates, family and adoption studies support a monogenic autosomal dominant basis, with low penetrance. Gene mapping indicates genetic heterogeneity.

Suggested environmental triggers include prenatal viral infection and social stress.

## Affective disorder

**Affective disorders** include purely **depressive** or **unipolar,** and **manic depressive** or **bipolar illness**. The average lifetime risk for bipolar is about 1%, for unipolar 2–25% depending on cultural background.

Twin, family and adoption studies point to a genetic basis. Mapping studies indicate genetic heterogeneity and there is evidence of anticipation, possibly indicative of an unstable triplet repeat (see Chapters 29 and 30).

## Alzheimer disease

**Alzheimer disease** involves **dementia** (progressive impairment of intellect, etc.) in 10% of those over 65 years, increasing to 50% at 80 years. It is also a feature of Down syndrome (see Chapter 14).

In families with early onset disease dominant inheritance is indicated, with at least seven susceptibility loci, including **presenilin-1** and **presenilin-2**, and environmental risk factors. Late onset cases fit a multifactorial model best, with the **epsilon 4 ($\varepsilon$4)** allele of **apolipoprotein E** as the best characterized component.

## Others

**Multiple sclerosis**, **rheumatoid arthritis** and many other conditions have major genetic and environmental components and notable associations with the human leucocyte antigen (HLA) system (see Chapter 27). Twin concordance rates for **tuberculosis** and **leprosy**, as distinct from those for **measles**, also reveal genetic components.

**Table 23.2** Relative risk and degree of relationship for some common diseases.

| Frequency in relatives (%) | | | |
| --- | --- | --- | --- |
| Disorder | First degree | Second degree | Third degree |
| Epilepsy | 5 | 2.5 | 1.5 |
| Schizophrenia | 10 | 4.0 | 2.0 |
| Bipolar affective disorder | 15 | 5.0 | 3.5 |

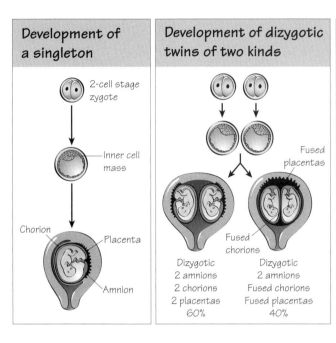

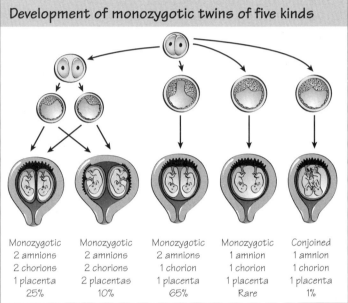

**Table 24.1** Twin concordance values for some developmental multifactorial threshold traits.

| Disorder | Frequency/1000 (Europeans) | MZ concordance (%) | DZ concordance (%) |
| --- | --- | --- | --- |
| Spina bifida | 5.0 | 6 | 3 |
| Talipes equinovarus | 5.0 | 32 | 3 |
| Pyloric stenosis | 3.0 | 15 | 2 |
| Congenital dislocation of the hip | 1.0 | 41 | 3 |
| Cleft lip ± palate | 1.0 | 30 | 5 |
| Cleft palate | 0.5 | 26 | 5 |

## Overview

The main value of twins in genetic analysis is that they can reveal the relative importance of genotype ('nature') and environment ('nurture') in multifactorial disease.

There are two major categories of twins, **monozygotic (MZ)** or **identical**, and **dizygotic (DZ)** or **fraternal**. DZ twins originate from two eggs and two sperm; like ordinary siblings they share 50% of their alleles. MZ twins originate from a single zygote that divided into two embryos during the first 2 weeks of development. MZ twins are always of the same sex and their genomes are 100% identical.

Sixty-five per cent of MZ twins share a placenta and chorion, around 25% have separate chorions and almost all have separate amnions. They have non-identical, but very similar, fingerprints. Their '**DNA fingerprints**' are identical (see Chapter 46).

## Frequency of multiple births

Around 1/80 British pregnancies yield twins, about 1/260 of MZ, 1/125 of DZ. Up to 1/20 births are of DZ in some African populations, but less than 1/500 in Chinese and Japanese. Multiple births involve various combinations of DZ- and MZ-like twinning events. Triplets occur in 1/7500 and quadruplets in 1/658 000 European births.

DZ twinning is increased at late births and greater maternal age, the peak being at age 35–40, possibly related to levels of **follicle stimulating hormone (FSH)**. Women treated with ovulation-inducing agents like *clomiphene citrate* and *gonadotrophins* are at increased risk of multiple pregnancy. There is probably no familial tendency toward MZ twinning, but there is for DZ, with up to three times the normal rate in some families.

## Analysis of discontinuous multifactorial traits

### Concordance ratio

If both twins are affected by a condition they are said to be **concordant** for that condition. If only one is affected they are **discordant**. The **pairwise concordance rate** is given by

$$C/(C + D)$$

where C = the number of concordant pairs and D = the number of discordant pairs.

Since MZ twins are genetically identical, whereas DZ share only 50% of their genomes, the ratio of their concordances for a condition gives a rough indication of the relative importance of genotype in its causation:

- If $C_{MZ} : C_{DZ} = 3\text{–}6 : 1$, the genome is the major determinant, e.g. schizophrenia, CL±P.
- If $C_{MZ} : C_{DZ} = 2\text{–}3 : 1$, both genetic and environmental factors are significant, e.g. blood pressure, mental deficiency.
- If $C_{MZ} : C_{DZ} = 1\text{–}2 : 1$, the main determinant is environmental, e.g. measles, tobacco smoking.

### The Holzinger statistic

The Holzinger ($H$) statistic provides values from close to zero, for minimal genetic involvement, to close to unity for almost entirely genetic causation:

$$H = \frac{C_{MZ} - C_{DZ}}{1 - C_{DZ}}$$

### Estimation of penetrance and gene counting

MZ concordance relates to penetrance ($P$) by the expression:

$$C_{MZ} = \frac{P}{2 - P},$$

from which penetrance can be calculated.

When $P$ is known the number of major causative alleles can be derived from DZ concordance:

$$C_{DZ} = \frac{P}{4 - P}, \text{ for ONE major autosomal dominant;}$$

$$C_{DZ} = \frac{P}{8 - P}, \text{ for TWO dominants, or a pair of recessives;}$$

$$C_{DZ} = \frac{P}{16 - P}, \text{ for THREE dominants, or one dominant and a pair of}$$
recessives.

## Analysis of continuously variable multifactorial traits

The most widely used estimate of genetic involvement is **heritability** ($h^2$), defined as *the fraction of variation in a quantitative character that can be ascribed to genotypic variation*. It can furnish information on, for example, the effectiveness of a nutritional regime. It applies to populations, not individuals and varies between populations.

Heritability is derivable from several kinds of data, including the standard deviations of the differences between cotwins, or the coefficients of correlation between them.

### From standard deviations

'Variation' is equated with 'variance', the square of the standard deviation of the differences between members of twin pairs:

$$h^2 = \frac{V_{DZ} - V_{MZ}}{V_{DZ}}$$

### From correlation coefficients ($r$)

$$h^2 = \frac{r_{MZ} - r_{DZ}}{1 - r_{DZ}}$$

## Health risks in twins

Twin pregnancies have a 5–10-fold increased incidence of perinatal mortality and a tendency toward premature birth. Due to crowding, *in utero* deformations occur in both kinds of twins, but MZ pregnancies are also associated with twice the normal risk of malformation (see Chapter 21).

Monochorionic MZ twins may (~15%) share a blood supply. This can lead to **twin-to-twin transfusion syndrome** when one twin becomes severely undernourished while the other develops an enlarged heart and liver and **polyhydramnios** (excessive amniotic fluid; see Chapter 21). There are marked differences in birth weights and both twins are at great risk of morbidity and mortality.

## Conjoined twins

**Conjoined**, or 'Siamese' **twins** develop from incompletely separated inner-cell masses and occur in about 1% of MZ pairs. They may be united at any part of the head or trunk but at the same position on each individual.

## Parasitic twins

A parasitic twin is a portion of a body protruding from an otherwise normal host. Common attachment sites are the oral region, the pelvis and the **mediastinum** (the wall dividing the thoracic cavity).

## Vanishing twins

Early loss and partial or complete resorption of one member of a twin pair is not unusual and can cause discrepancy between prenatal and postnatal cytogenetic findings.

## Reversed asymmetry

Asymmetric anatomical features sometimes show reversal in one twin. This is especially so in conjoined pairs and in those MZ twin pairs that result from late division.

## Problems of twin studies

**1** Concordant pairs can be **ascertained** (i.e. recognized) through both individuals, discordant through only one, leading to **bias of ascertainment**.
**2** The first two division products of an oocyte may be fertilized by separate sperms.
**3** There may be coincident fertilization of separate eggs by different fathers.
**4** MZ discordance can arise from somatic mutation or transfusion syndrome, rather than incomplete penetrance.

# 25 Normal polymorphism

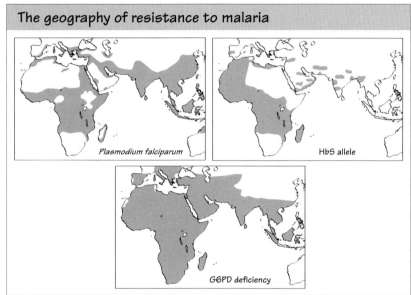

The geography of resistance to malaria

*Plasmodium falciparum*

HbS allele

G6PD deficiency

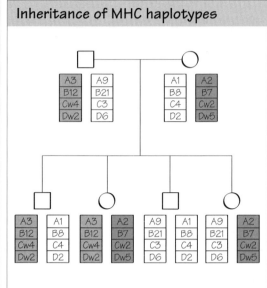

Inheritance of MHC haplotypes

## Overview

**Genetic polymorphism** is the occurrence of multiple alleles at a locus, where at least two are at frequencies greater than 1%. Over 30% of structural genes are polymorphic. Part III deals with their application at the DNA level.

## Environment-related polymorphism
### Sunlight

Skin colour relates to the prevailing intensity of sunlight in the region of origin of a population. Sunburn, skin cancer and toxic accumulation of vitamin D select for dark skin in sunny climates. Deficiency of vitamin D selects for pale skin in less sunny regions, by causing **rickets**, formerly lethal to women at childbirth.

### Food

Worldwide, most human adults cannot tolerate **lactose**, but traditional consumption of cows' milk has selected lactose tolerance in Europeans and in some North Africans. Australian aborigines readily become hypertensive if they consume common salt. Other foods cause health problems for carriers of specific polymorphic variants (see Chapter 47).

### Alcohol

Ethyl alcohol is metabolized to acetaldehyde by **alcohol dehydrogenase (ADH)**, of which there are several types. Ninety per cent of Chinese and Japanese people, and 5% of British people have a deficient form of ADH2, making them more prone to intoxication.

Acetaldehyde is further degraded by cytosolic **acetaldehyde dehydrogenase 1 (ALDH1)** and mitochondrial **ALDH2**. Up to 50% of Asians are deficient in ALDH2 and experience an unpleasant **'flushing'** reaction to alcohol caused by accumulation of acetaldehyde.

## Malaria
### Sickle cell anaemia (intermediate dominance)

The **HbS** allele of β-globin causes reduced solubility of haemoglobin in homozygotes (*HbS/HbS*), and their red blood corpuscles collapse, characteristically into a sickle shape, when oxygen concentrations are low. The 'sickled cells' clog capillaries causing death in childhood (see Chapters 19 and 30).

Heterozygotes (*HbS/HbA*) have **'the sickle cell trait'**. In low oxygen regimes they suffer capillary blockage, but they have the great advantage of resistance to the malaria parasite, *Plasmodium falciparum*. By eliminating normal homozygotes (*HbA/HbA*) malaria creates high frequencies of the HbS allele in malarial areas (see figure).

Sickle cell disease is the classic example of a **balanced polymorphism**.

### Thalassaemia (recessive)

**Thalassaemia** is a quantitative or functional deficiency of **α-,** or **β-globin** (see Chapter 30 and Tables 25.1 and 25.2 ). Homozygosity of some alleles is lethal, but heterozygosity of beta-thalassaemia and alpha-thalassaemia trait (or type 2) afford protection in malarial areas around the Mediterranean Sea, the Middle East and South-East Asia.

**Table 25.1** Genetic bases of alpha-thalassaemia.

| Phenotype | Genotype | Quantity of α-globin produced (%) |
|---|---|---|
| Normal | $\alpha\alpha/\alpha\alpha$ | 100 |
| 'Silent carrier' | $\alpha-/\alpha\alpha$ | 75 |
| 'Alpha-thalassaemia trait' | $\alpha-/\alpha-$ or $--/\alpha\alpha$ | 50 |
| Haemoglobin H (β4) | $\alpha-/--$ | 25 |
| Hydrops foetalis | $--/--$ | 0 (lethal) |

**Table 25.2** Genetic bases of beta-thalassaemia.

| Affected population | Nature of defect | β-globin phenotype |
|---|---|---|
| Italian | δ/β fusion protein | β° |
| Sardinian | premature termination | β° |
| African | RNA splicing | β° |
| | RNA splicing | β+ |
| | polyadenylation | β+ |
| Japanese | promoter | β+ |
| Indian | deletion | β° |
| | frameshift + premature termination | β° |
| Asian | mRNA capping | β+ |
| South-East Asian | substitution | β+ |

*Glucose-6-phosphate dehydrogenase deficiency (X-linked recessive)*

Deficiency of **glucose-6-phosphate dehydrogenase** (G6PD) is very common in malarial areas (see figure) as it prevents growth of *Plasmodium* parasites. This advantage is confined to females.

*The Duffy blood group (codominant)*

There are three alleles of the **Duffy blood group**, $Fy^A$, $Fy^B$ and $Fy^O$, the latter reaching 100% frequency in some African populations. $Fy^A$ and $Fy^B$ provide an entry gate for malaria parasites into red cells, but $Fy^O$ does not, so making homozygotes resistant.

## Transfusion and transplantation
### The ABO system

The ABO blood groups (see Chapter 19) are a vital consideration in blood transfusion and tissue transplantation because we naturally carry antibodies directed against those antigens we do not ourselves possess (Table 25.3).

Group O are **universal donors**, Group AB **universal recipients**.

**Table 25.3** Transfusion relations between the ABO blood groups.

| Blood group | UK frequency* | Antigens on RBCs | Antibodies in serum | Can receive from | Can donate to |
|---|---|---|---|---|---|
| A | 0.42 | A | Anti-B | A or O | A or AB |
| B | 0.09 | B | Anti-A | B or O | B or AB |
| AB | 0.03 | A+B | None | **Everyone** | AB only |
| O | 0.46 | None | Anti-A + anti-B | O only | **Everyone** |

RBCs, red blood cells.
*Allele frequencies vary widely between populations.

### The Rhesus system

The Rhesus system is genetically complex, but can be considered as involving two alleles, *D* and *d*. *DD* and *Dd* individuals display Rhesus antigens on their red cells and are said to be **Rhesus positive (Rh+)**. Rh+ individuals can be given Rh- blood, but **Rh- (*dd*)** individuals develop an immune response if transfused with Rh+ blood.

If a Rh- woman is pregnant with a Rh+ (*Dd*) baby she can become immunized against red blood cells that leak across the placenta. Anti-Rh antibodies can then invade the baby causing **haemolytic disease of the newborn**.

### The major histocompatibility complex (HLA) system

The **MHC**, or **HLA system** contains three classes of genes concerned with the immune response (see Chapter 33). Class I includes HLA-A (23 alleles), HLA-B (47 alleles) and HLA-C (eight alleles); Class II, HLA-DP (six alleles), -DQ (three alleles) and -DR (14 alleles). Since their products are potent antigens and highly polymorphic, there are serious problems of compatibility in organ transplantation. The chance of a random HLA match is about 1/200 000.

The MHC loci are closely linked and usually transmitted together as a **haplotype**. There is a 25% chance that two sibs inherit matching HLA haplotypes or, if parents share a haplotype, a similar chance of a match between parent and offspring (see figure).

## Pharmacogenetics
### G6PD deficiency (X-linked recessive)

G6PD deficiency causes sensitivity to some drugs, notably **primaquine** (used for treatment of malaria), **phenacetin**, **sulphonamides** and **fava beans** (broad beans), hence the name 'favism' for the haemolytic crisis that occurs when they are eaten (usually by males).

### N-acetyl transferase deficiency (recessive)

Fifty per cent of members of Western populations are homozygous for a recessive allele that confers a dangerously slow rate of elimination of certain drugs, notably **isoniazid** prescribed against tuberculosis. The Japanese are predominantly rapid inactivators.

### Pseudocholinesterase deficiency (recessive)

One European in 3000 and 1.5% of Inuit (Eskimo) are homozygous for an enzyme deficiency that causes lethal paralysis of the diaphragm when given **succinylcholine** as a muscle relaxant during surgery.

### Halothane sensitivity, malignant hyperthermia (genetically heterogeneous)

One in 10 000 patients dies in high fever when given the anaesthetic **halothane**, especially in combination with succinylcholine.

### Thiopurine methyltransferase deficiency (autosomal codominant)

Certain drugs prescribed for leukaemia and suppression of the immune response cause serious side-effects in about 0.3% of the population with deficiency of **thiopurine methyltransferase.**

### Debrisoquine hydroxylase deficiency (autosomal recessive)

This is one of the large P450 group important in deactivation of many drugs. Five to 10% of Europeans show serious adverse reactions when given **debrisoquine** for hypertension.

### Porphyria variegata (dominant)

Skin lesions, abdominal pain, paralysis, dementia and psychosis are brought on by sulphonamides, barbiturates, etc. It affects about one in 500 South Africans.

## Diallelic autosomal system with codominance, the MN blood groups

Proportions of genotypes in 100 zygotes obtained by 'random fertilization'.

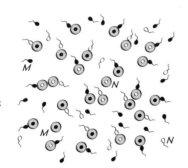

$M$-carrying cells are represented with black nuclei; $N$-carrying with white. Frequency of $M$ alleles = $p$ = 0.6; frequency of $N$ alleles = $q$ = 0.4

Geometric representation of the Hardy–Weinberg law applied to the $MN$ blood group system

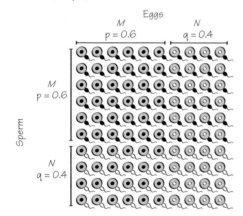

|  | Eggs | |
|---|---|---|
| Allele frequencies (total 1.0) | $M$ $p$ = 0.6 | $N$ $q$ = 0.4 |
| **Sperm** $M$ $p$ = 0.6 | $MM$ $p^2$ = 0.6 × 0.6 = 0.36 or 36% Homozygotes | $MN$ $pq$ = 0.6 × 0.4 = 0.24 or 24% Heterozygotes |
| $N$ $q$ = 0.4 | $MN$ $pq$ = 0.6 × 0.4 = 0.24 or 24% Heterozygotes | $NN$ $q^2$ = 0.4 × 0.4 = 0.16 or 16% Homozygotes |

Total $MN$ = 2$pq$ = 48%

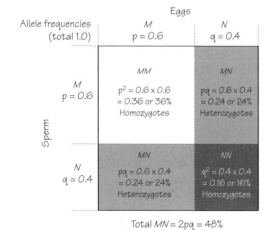

## Diallelic autosomal system with dominance and recessivity, albinism

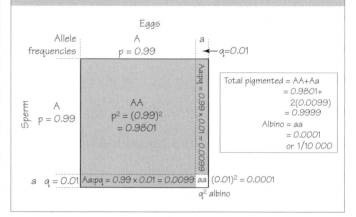

|  | Eggs | |
|---|---|---|
| Allele frequencies | A $p$ = 0.99 | a ← $q$ = 0.01 |
| **Sperm** A $p$ = 0.99 | AA $p^2$ = $(0.99)^2$ = 0.9801 | Aa:$pq$ = 0.99 × 0.01 = 0.0099 |
| a $q$ = 0.01 | Aa:$pq$ = 0.99 × 0.01 = 0.0099 | aa $(0.01)^2$ = 0.0001 $q^2$ albino |

Total pigmented = AA+Aa
= 0.9801+
2(0.0099)
= 0.9999
Albino = aa
= 0.0001
or 1/10 000

## Triallelic autosomal system with codominance and dominance, the ABO blood groups

(These frequencies are imaginary, see Chapter 25 for real values)

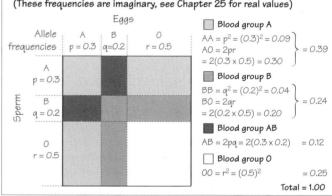

|  | Eggs | | |
|---|---|---|---|
| Allele frequencies | A $p$ = 0.3 | B $q$ = 0.2 | O $r$ = 0.5 |
| **Sperm** A $p$ = 0.3 | | | |
| B $q$ = 0.2 | | | |
| O $r$ = 0.5 | | | |

■ Blood group A
AA = $p^2$ = $(0.3)^2$ = 0.09
AO = 2$pr$
= 2(0.3 × 0.5) = 0.30 } = 0.39

■ Blood group B
BB = $q^2$ = $(0.2)^2$ = 0.04
BO = 2$qr$
= 2(0.2 × 0.5) = 0.20 } = 0.24

■ Blood group AB
AB = 2$pq$ = 2(0.3 × 0.2) = 0.12

□ Blood group O
OO = $r^2$ = $(0.5)^2$ = 0.25

Total = 1.00

## Relative frequency of recessive homozygotes and heterozygotes for some important recessive diseases

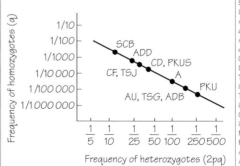

SCB, sickle cell anaemia in US black people
ADD, α1-antitrypsin deficiency in US black people
ADB, α1-antitrypsin deficiency in Denmark
CF, cystic fibrosis in US white people
TSJ, Tay–Sachs disease in US Ashkenasi Jews
TSG, Tay–Sachs disease in US non-white Jews
CD, congenital deafness in the US
PKUS, phenylketonuria in Finland, Japan and the Jews
A, albinism in the US
AU, alcaptonuria in the US

## Overview

Within a *randomly mating* population the relative frequencies of heterozygotes and homozygotes are mathematically related to allele frequencies by what is known as the **Hardy–Weinberg law**. Extension of this theory reveals that *allele frequencies will remain constant from generation to generation provided none is under positive or negative selection*. This is the 'Hardy–Weinberg equilibrium'.

## The Hardy–Weinberg law
### Diallelic autosomal system with codominance
In the **MN blood group system** alleles **M** and **N** are codominant and there are three blood groups: **M**, **MN** and **N**, M and N individuals being homozygotes. We can calculate the frequency ($p$) of allele **M** in a population as the proportion of group M individuals plus half the proportion of group MN. Similarly, the frequency ($q$) of allele **N** equals the proportion of group N people plus half the proportion of group MN. Since there are no other alleles, $p + q = 1$. If Hardy–Weinberg conditions apply the frequencies of the genotypes are given by: $(p + q)^2 = p^2 + 2pq + q^2$, i.e. frequency of $MM = p^2$, frequency of $MN = 2pq$ and frequency of $NN = q^2$.

### Diallelic autosomal system with dominance and recessivity (e.g. albinism)
If the frequency of a dominant allele $A$ is $p$ and that of a recessive allele $a$ at the same locus is $q$ and there are no other alleles, then the frequencies of the genotypes are $AA$, $p^2$; $Aa$, $2pq$; $aa$, $q^2$. The frequencies of the phenotypes are **pigmented**: $p^2 + 2pq$; **albino**: $q^2$.

### Triallelic autosomal system with codominance and dominance (e.g. the ABO blood groups)
If the population frequencies of alleles $A$, $B$ and $O$ are $p$, $q$ and $r$, respectively, then $p + q + r = 1$ and the frequencies of the genotypes, from $(p + q + r)^2$, are $AA$, $p^2$; $BB$, $q^2$; $OO$, $r^2$; $AB$, $2pq$; $AO$, $2pr$; $BO$, $2qr$. The frequencies of the blood groups are **A**: $p^2 + 2pr$; **B**: $q^2 + 2qr$; **O**: $r^2$; and **AB**: $2pq$.

### Diallelic X-linked system with dominance and recessivity (e.g. G6PD deficiency)
If the frequency of allele $G$ is $p$ and that of allele $g$ is $q$, then the frequency of **G** phenotype males is $p$ and that of **g** phenotype males is $q$. In females the frequencies of the genotypes are: $GG$, $p^2$; $Gg$, $2pq$; $gg$, $q^2$, and the frequencies of the phenotypes are **G**, $p^2 + 2pq$; **g**, $q^2$.

## Necessary conditions
1  **Random mating**. Two conditions can lead to over-representation of homozygotes: (i) **assortative mating**: usually selection of a mate on the basis of similarity with self, e.g. for deafness, stature, religion or ethnicity; and (ii) **consanguinity**, e.g. cousin marriage. Homozygosity exposes disadvantageous recessives to selection, which may alter their frequency in subsequent generations.
2  **Absence of selection**, i.e. no genotypic class may be less or more viable than the others. Allowance must therefore be made for disease alleles.
3  **Lack of relevant mutation**.
4  **Large population size**. In small populations random fluctuations in gene frequency (**genetic drift**) can result in **extinction** of some alleles, **fixation** of others.
5  **Absence of gene flow**. Migration of people slowly spreads variant alleles. An example is indicated by the cline in blood group B from 0.3 in East Asia to 0.06 in Western Europe.

## Applications of the Hardy–Weinberg law

These include:
1  Recognition of reduced viability of certain genotypes.
2  Estimation of the probability of finding a specific tissue antigen match in the general population.
3  Estimation of the number of potential donors of a rare blood group.
4  Estimation of the frequency of carriers of autosomal recessive disease. *The frequency of unaffected heterozygotes is invariably very much higher than that of affected recessive homozygotes* (see figure).

## Examples
### Autosomal recessive conditions
*Phenylketonuria*
Phenylketonuria occurs in US whites at a frequency of ~1/15 000. What is the frequency of heterozygous carriers?
Homozygote frequency, $q^2 = 1/15\,000$;
disease allele frequency, $q = \sqrt{1/15\,000} = 0.008$;
normal allele frequency, $p = 1 - q = 1 - 0.008 = 0.992$.
**Heterozygote frequency, $2pq = 2 \times 0.992 \times 0.008 = 0.016 = 1.6\%$ or ~1/60**.

*Cystic fibrosis*
Cystic fibrosis occurs in US whites at a frequency of ~1/2500. What is the frequency of marriages (at random) between cystic fibrosis heterozygotes?
$q^2 = 1/2500$;
$q = \sqrt{1/2500} = 1/50 = 0.02$;
$p = 1 - q = 1 - 0.02 = 0.98$;
carrier frequency $= 2pq = 2 \times 0.98 \times 0.02 = 0.04$.
**Frequency of marriages between heterozygotes $= (2pq)^2 = (0.04)^2 = 0.0016$ or 0.16%**.

### X-linked recessive conditions
*Haemophilia A*
Haemophilia A occurs in 1/5000 male births. What is the frequency of female carriers?
$q = $ frequency of disease in males $= 1/5000 = 0.0002$;
$p = 1 - q = 1 - 0.0002 = 0.9998$.
**Frequency of female carriers $= 2pq = 2 \times 0.9998 \times 0.0002 = 0.0004 = 0.04\%$, or 1/2500**.

*Colour blindness*
Colour blindness is present in 8% of British males. What is the frequency of affected females?
Colour blindness allele frequency $= q = 0.08$.
**Frequency of affected females $= q^2 = (0.08)^2 = 0.0064 = 0.64\%$ or 1/156**.

## Consequences of medical intervention
When medical intervention introduces major improvements in the biological fitness of carriers of lethal or seriously disabling alleles, this has serious effects on allele frequency. For example, one-third of all copies of X-linked disease alleles are in males. A major increase in the survival or fertility of male hemizygotes can therefore increase disease frequency by up to 33% *per generation*. Medical intervention can *double* the frequency of serious autosomal dominant disease *at each successive generation*. Recessive disease frequency could theoretically *quadruple* in 1/q generations; e.g. if q = 1/25, in 25 generations (see Chapter 34).

# 27 Genetic linkage and disease association

## Pedigree showing linkage of the nail–patella gene locus with the ABO blood group locus

In most individuals the dominant disease allele Np is in coupling with the B allele

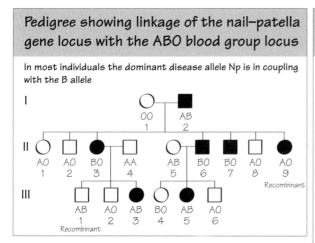

## Characteristic posture of a patient with ankylosing spondylitis (very strongly associated with HLA-B27)

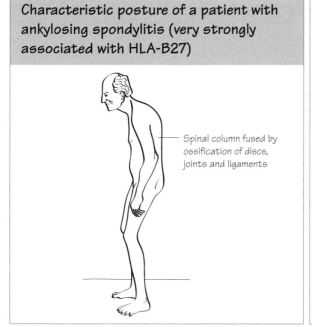

Spinal column fused by ossification of discs, joints and ligaments

## Crossing over between homologous chromosomes in meiosis

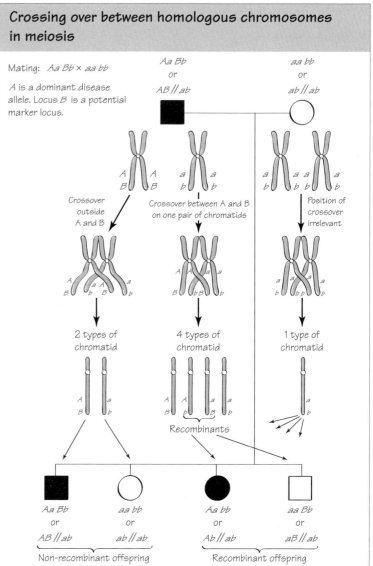

Mating: $Aa\,Bb \times aa\,bb$

$A$ is a dominant disease allele. Locus $B$ is a potential marker locus.

## Overview

**Genetic linkage** is the tendency for alleles close together on the same chromosome to be transmitted together to offspring. It is of very great value in genetic prognosis (Chapter 42).

**Disease association** is the appearance in many patients of a second genetically determined character at a frequency higher than would be predicted on the basis of their independent frequencies. In a few cases this involves **linkage disequilibrium**, but in most it does not.

A group of disease features that regularly occur together, usually due to pleiotropic expression of one allele, is called a **syndrome**. Distinction between a syndrome and the effects of linked genes involves: (i) *deducing a logical causal relationship between the features*; or (ii) *discovering instances where the frequently associated characters do* not *occur together*.

## Genetic linkage

Assume two loci, *A* and *B*, are close together on the same chromosome and we observe 'test matings' of type (i) *AB//ab×ab//ab*, or type (ii) *Ab//aB×ab//ab,* where / represents a chromosome. In type (i) matings, dominant alleles *A* and *B* are on the same chromosome and recessive alleles *a* and *b* on its homologue. The dominants and recessives are said to be '**in coupling**', or *cis* to one another. In matings of type (ii) the dominant and recessive alleles on opposite chromosomes are '**in repulsion**', or *trans* to one another.

Since loci A and B are close, chiasmata rarely occur between them and the parental combinations *AB* and *ab*, or *Ab* and *aB,* will be more frequently represented among offspring than the recombinant combinations *Ab* and *aB*, or *AB, ab*, respectively.

Gregor Mendel was unaware of linkage and according to his principle of Independent Assortment (see Chapter 16), all four types of offspring: *AaBb*, *Aabb*, *aaBb* and *aabb* should be equally represented. When they are not, this is evidence of linkage.

If an allele of gene *A* causes disease, but is otherwise undetectable, whereas the alleles of gene *B* can be easily detected and distinguished, gene *B* can be used as a marker for the inherited disease. This is not completely reliable, as crossover occasionally occurs between them. For accurate prediction we need to know the **crossover frequency**, i.e. we need to 'map' their relative positions. A marker locus five **map units** from a disease gene segregates from it in 5% of meioses, so predictions based on that marker are accurate in 95% of cases.

Historically important linkages are of ABO to **nail–patella syndrome** and of **secretor** to **myotonic dystrophy**. Currently the most useful markers are **microsatellite DNA** variants (see Part III).

## Gene mapping

The genetic **map distance** between loci *A* and *B* can be deduced from the frequency of recombination between them, by the formula:

$$\frac{\text{Number of recombinant offspring} \times 100}{\text{Total number of offspring}}$$

i.e. in type i) matings:
$$\frac{(Aabb + aaBb) \times 100}{Aabb + aaBb + AaBb + aabb}$$

Or, in type ii):
$$\frac{(AaBb + aabb) \times 100}{Aabb + aaBb + AaBb + aabb}$$

The unit of map distance is the **centiMorgan (cM)** and *map distances derived in this way never exceed 50 cM*, as this corresponds to independent assortment, i.e. non-linkage.

Longer distances can be mapped by adding together the map distances between intermediate loci.

A gene map constructed from crossovers in males gives the same gene order as one constructed from crossovers in females, but the calculated 'distances' between them are often different. This is because chiasmata occur at different frequencies in the formation of ova and sperm. There are also 'hot spots' of high recombination frequency on some chromosomes.

The total map length of the genome, estimated from visible chiasmata in primary germ cells, is ~3000 cM in males and ~4200 cM in females. Since the haploid *physical* length of the genome is about 3000 million bp, 1 cM corresponds to about a million base pairs in males, and 700 000 in females.

Additional techniques of gene mapping and its diagnostic applications are discussed in Chapters 28 and 42.

## LOD score analysis

The reliability of a suspected linkage can be confirmed by 'LOD score analysis' of family pedigrees. The word LOD is derived from 'log of the odds', the logarithm ($\log_{10}$) of the ratio of the probability that the observed ratio of offspring arose as a result of genetic linkage (of specified degree) to the probability that it arose merely by chance.

The **maximum LOD score** is the total value of the combined LODs, usually for a group of families, calculated at the most probable degree of linkage. A *value that exceeds +3 is accepted as evidence favouring autosomal linkage (or of +2 for linkage on the X); one of less than –2, of non-linkage.*

## Disease association

Many of the most important disease associations involve the HLA system. For example, more than 90% of individuals with the connective tissue disease **ankylosing spondylitis** (AS, or 'poker spine') carry a specific HLA allele, namely HLA-B27. AS is a chronic inflammatory condition of the spine and sacro-iliac joints that leads to their fusion. Five per cent of Europeans have HLA-B27 and, although only 1% of these actually has AS, their 'risk' is considered to be 90 times as high as those who are B27-negative. This association of HLA-B27 with AS is believed to involve interference in the generation of an immune response specifically to infection by the bacterium *Klebsiella*.

There are many other HLA-associated diseases, most of which do not involve linkage to the MHC (see Chapter 23). **Primary haemochromatosis** and **congenital adrenal hyperplasia** are exceptions which show **linkage disequilibrium** with specific HLA haplotypes. Linkage disequilibrium exists because the disease alleles arose on very few occasions and have not yet segregated from their original haplotypes.

Most other cases, including AS, involve **auto-immunity**, i.e. there is an immune response directed apparently against self-antigens (see Chapters 23 and 33).

**Table 27.1** Important HLA associations of some common diseases.

| HLA | Disease | Frequency in patients (%) | Frequency in general pop. (%) | Relative risk* |
|---|---|---|---|---|
| A3 | Haemochromatosis | 75 | 13 | 20 |
| B17 | Psoriasis | 38 | 8 | 7 |
| B27 | Ankylosing spondylitis | >90 | 8 | >100 |
| | Reiter syndrome | 75 | 8 | 35 |
| B47 | Congenital adrenal hyperplasia | 17 | 0.4 | 51 |
| Cw6 | Psoriasis | >50 | 9 | >10 |
| DR2 | Narcolepsy | ~100 | 16 | >100 |
| | Goodpasture syndrome | 88 | 32 | 16 |
| | Multiple sclerosis | 57 | 21 | 5 |
| | Systemic lupus erythematosus | >70 | 16 | >12 |
| DR3 | Systemic lupus erythematosus | 50 | 25 | 3 |
| | Coeliac disease | 60 | 12 | 11 |
| | IDDM | 50 | 12 | 7 |
| DR4 | IDDM | 38 | 13 | 4 |
| DR3//DR4 | IDDM | | | 33 |
| DR5 | Juvenile rheumatoid arthritis | 50 | 16 | 5 |
| | Pernicious anaemia | 25 | 6 | 5 |

HLA, human leucocyte antigen; IDDM, insulin dependent diabetes mellitus.
*Relative risk = ad/bc, where a = number of patients with the antigen, b = number of controls with the antigen, c = number of patients without the antigen and d = number of controls without the antigen.

## The positional cloning approach to gene mapping and defect characterization

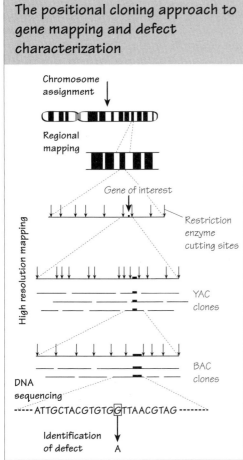

Chromosome assignment

Regional mapping

Gene of interest

Restriction enzyme cutting sites

High resolution mapping

YAC clones

BAC clones

DNA sequencing

----- ATTGCTACGTGTG**G**TTAACGTAG --------

Identification of defect

A

## Multipoint mapping

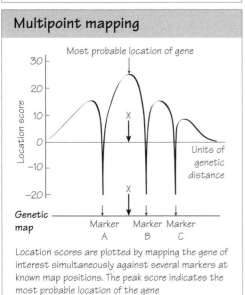

Most probable location of gene

Location score

Units of genetic distance

Genetic map

Marker A    Marker B    Marker C

Location scores are plotted by mapping the gene of interest simultaneously against several markers at known map positions. The peak score indicates the most probable location of the gene

## Chromosome flow sorting

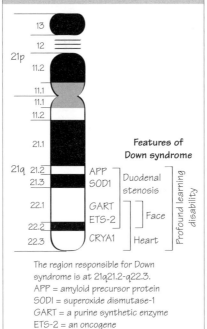

Metaphase chromosome preparation

UV laser

Fluorescence sensor

Charging collar

Computer

Deflecting plates

++    +

Chromosomes fractionated on the basis of charge

## Phenotypic map of Trisomy 21, based on individuals with partial trisomies

13
12
21p
11.2
11.1
11.1
11.2
21.1
21q   21.2    APP ⎫
      21.3    SOD1 ⎬ Duodenal stenosis
      22.1    GART ⎫
              ETS-2 ⎬ Face
      22.2
      22.3    CRYA1 ⎦ Heart

Features of Down syndrome

Profound learning disability

The region responsible for Down syndrome is at 21q21.2–q22.3.
APP = amyloid precursor protein
SODI = superoxide dismutase-1
GART = a purine synthetic enzyme
ETS-2 = an oncogene
CRYA1 = alpha crystallin

## Crossover analysis with flanking markers

A
B
C
D
E
F

Known order of markers

Haplotypes are shown for markers A–F known to map to the same region as the disease gene. Analysis shows the gene to map between markers B and C

## Table 28.1 Approaches for physical gene mapping

An average gene occupies about 1000 bp (1 kb) (1 cM is about $10^6$ bp [1 Mb]). An average chromosome is about 150 cM or 150 Mb

| Basis of method | Goal | Resolution (base pairs) |
|---|---|---|
| Somatic cell hybrids Flow cytometry | Chromosome assignment | $50–250 \times 10^6$ |
| Chromosome rearrangements Gene dosage analysis Cross-over analysis | Regional mapping | $5–20 \times 10^6$ |
| In situ hybridization Linkage analysis Restriction mapping Chromosome walking | Fine-scale mapping | $10^5–10^6$ |
| Cloning in YACs Cloning in BACs DNA sequencing | Large-scale cloning Gene cloning Nucleotide sequence | $10^5–10^6$ $10^{3-5} \times 10^4$ 1 |

BACs, bacterial artificial chromosomes
YACs, yeast artificial chromosomes

## Overview

There are two fundamentally different approaches to mapping human genes: **genetic mapping** involves measurement of the tendency of genes to cosegregate through meiosis; **physical mapping** deals with the assignment of genes to specific physical locations. **The Human Genome Project** aims to produce a complete gene map and record of the entire nucleotide sequence of the human genome by the year 2003.

Gene mapping exercises generally progress through four stages:

1 chromosome assignment;
2 regional mapping;
3 high-resolution mapping;
4 DNA sequencing (see Chapter 43).

## Chromosome assignment
### Patterns of transmission

Five locations are indicated by characteristic patterns of transmission. These are autosomal, X and Y, pseudo-autosomal and mitochondrial (see Chapters 17–20).

### Chromosome flow-sorting or flow cytometry

A culture of dividing cells is arrested at metaphase and the chromosomes released and stained with a fluorescent DNA stain. The preparation is then squirted through a fine jet, vertically downwards through a UV laser beam. As each chromosome fluoresces it acquires an electrical charge and is deflected by an electrical potential across its path. Deflection is proportional to intensity of fluorescence and this allows preparations of individual chomosomes to be amassed.

Such chromosome preparations can be used for making chromosome paints (see Chapter 38 and book cover) or chromosome-specific 'dot-blots' on nitrocellulose membranes. Sequences can then be assigned to chromosomes merely by testing their capacity to hybridize with the dot-blots (see Chapter 44).

### Somatic cell hybrids

A **somatic cell hybrid** is produced by fusing together two somatic cells or by incorporating a foreign genome into a cell. By careful selection, cloning and long-term maintenance it is possible to create cultures of mouse–human cells containing a single human chromosome along with most of the mouse genome. Chromosome assignment of the genes for human proteins synthesized in such cultures is then a matter of recognizing the human chromosome present.

## Regional mapping
### Family linkage studies

The frequency of cross-over between loci relates inversely to the physical distance between them by a mathematical expression called **the mapping function.**

Autosomal traits have been assigned to chromosomes on the basis of cotransmission with cytogenetic features such as translocation breakpoints, or linkage to already assigned markers, an early objective being the identification of DNA markers at 10 cM intervals throughout the genome (see Chapter 27).

When many loci are involved, advanced computer programs can integrate linkage data in 'multipoint maps', to produce 'locations scores' (c.f. LOD scores for single genes; see Chapter 27).

### Restriction mapping

DNA is digested with a restriction enzyme and subjected to electrophoresis, etc., as described for Southern blotting (see Chapter 44). By use of several enzymes that cleave DNA at different sites, and recognizing regions of overlap between different fragments, we can map the enzyme-susceptible sites, and order the fragments.

### Cross-over analysis

This approach aims to map a gene by defining its haplotype with respect to adjacent markers before and after cross-over (see figure).

### Gene dosage

Normally every individual has two copies of every autosomal gene. Exceptions include heterozygotes for a deletion and trisomics. Among these, the amount of primary gene product can vary three-fold. The location of a gene can sometimes be determined by relating quantity of enzyme to the chromosomal breakpoints.

### *In-situ* hybridization

The technique of FISH provides a spectacular approach to gene mapping (see Chapter 38). If a probe recognizes a specific gene sequence, both chromosomal and regional assignment is straightforward.

## High-resolution mapping
### Cloning

A range of advanced techniques, such as **chromosome microdissection**, **jumping** and **walking**, involve mass production of DNA fragments of a variety of lengths. Before PCR was developed (see Chapter 45) the only way to amplify a chosen gene sequence was by cloning in a microorganism. The basic idea is to insert the gene into a bacterial **plasmid** or **bacteriophage** and allow this to proliferate in a bacterial culture (see Chapter 44). Larger DNA fragments are cloned in artificial bacterial vectors called **cosmids** and **bacterial artificial chromosomes** (**BACs**), very large ones (50–1000 kb) in **yeast artificial chromosomes** (**YACs**).

### Fibre-FISH

Chromosomes are extended at interphase and this can be exploited to map genes by an adaptation of FISH called **fibre-FISH** or **DIRVISH** (**Dir**ect **Vis**ualization **H**ybridization). A liquid preparation of interphase DNA is applied to a microscope slide, which is tilted, causing the liquid to run down the slide and the chromosomes to become stretched along their lengths. Fluorescent probes directed against genes known to map to the same region are added to the slide and allowed to hybridize, when the order of the fluorescent signals indicates that of the genes along the chromosome.

## Two basic strategies for mapping genes

The **positional cloning approach** involves mapping the disease gene by conventional linkage analysis with respect to the nearest reliable marker.

An alternative is the **candidate gene approach**. In this, one identifies genes known to map to the indicated region or to have a role in relevant physiology. Patients are then screened for variants of these candidate genes. In both cases the gene is eventually isolated and the molecular defect(s) associated with disease deduced by sequencing (Chapter 43).

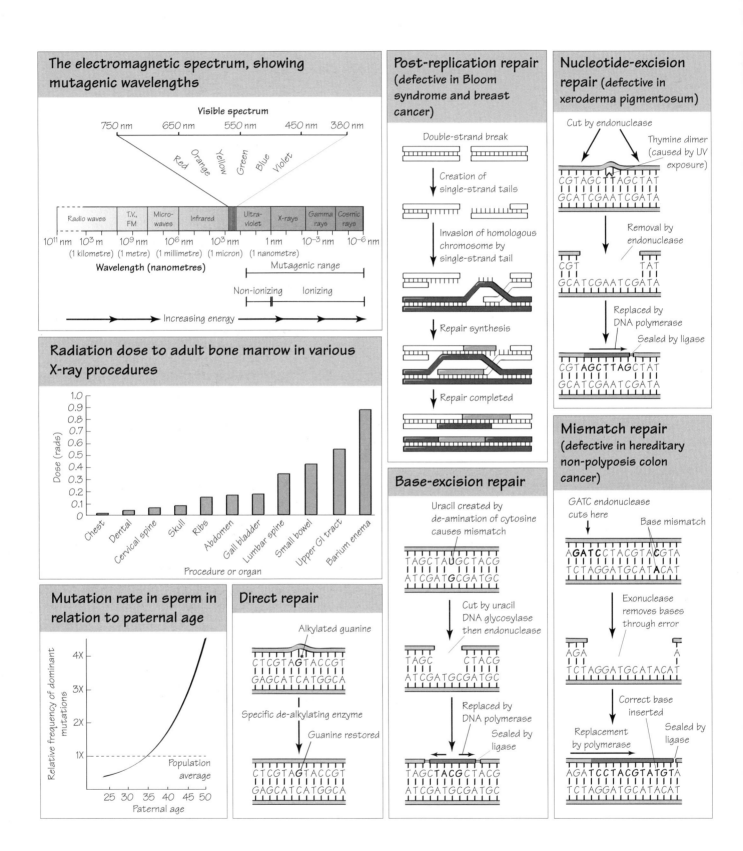

## The electromagnetic spectrum, showing mutagenic wavelengths

Visible spectrum

750 nm    650 nm    550 nm    450 nm    380 nm

Red  Orange  Yellow  Green  Blue  Violet

| Radio waves | T.V., FM | Micro-waves | Infrared | Ultra-violet | X-rays | Gamma rays | Cosmic rays |

$10^{11}$ nm   $10^3$ m   $10^9$ nm   $10^6$ nm   $10^3$ nm   1 nm   $10^{-3}$ nm   $10^{-6}$ nm

(1 kilometre) (1 metre) (1 millimetre) (1 micron) (1 nanometre)

Wavelength (nanometres)                    Mutagenic range

Non-ionizing    Ionizing

Increasing energy

## Radiation dose to adult bone marrow in various X-ray procedures

Dose (rads) — vertical axis from 0 to 1.0 in 0.1 increments

Procedure or organ: Chest, Dental, Cervical spine, Skull, Ribs, Abdomen, Gall bladder, Lumbar spine, Small bowel, Upper GI tract, Barium enema

## Mutation rate in sperm in relation to paternal age

Relative frequency of dominant mutations: 4X, 3X, 2X, 1X

Population average

Paternal age: 25 30 35 40 45 50

## Direct repair

Alkylated guanine

CTCGTAGTACCGT
GAGCATCATGGCA

Specific de-alkylating enzyme

Guanine restored

CTCGTAGTACCGT
GAGCATCATGGCA

## Post-replication repair (defective in Bloom syndrome and breast cancer)

Double-strand break

Creation of single-strand tails

Invasion of homologous chromosome by single-strand tail

Repair synthesis

Repair completed

## Base-excision repair

Uracil created by de-amination of cytosine causes mismatch

TAGCTAUGCTACG
ATCGATGCGATGC

Cut by uracil DNA glycosylase then endonuclease

TAGC    CTACG
ATCGATGCGATGC

Replaced by DNA polymerase
Sealed by ligase

TAGCTACGCTACG
ATCGATGCGATGC

## Nucleotide-excision repair (defective in xeroderma pigmentosum)

Cut by endonuclease

Thymine dimer (caused by UV exposure)

CGTAGCTTAGCTAT
GCATCGAATCGATA

Removal by endonuclease

CGT       TAT
GCATCGAATCGATA

Replaced by DNA polymerase
Sealed by ligase

CGTAGCTTAGCTAT
GCATCGAATCGATA

## Mismatch repair (defective in hereditary non-polyposis colon cancer)

GATC endonuclease cuts here

Base mismatch

AGATCCTACGTACGTA
TCTAGGATGCATACAT

Exonuclease removes bases through error

AGA          A
TCTAGGATGCATACAT

Correct base inserted

Replacement by polymerase
Sealed by ligase

AGATCCTACGTATGTA
TCTAGGATGCATACAT

## Overview

Apart from the effects of ultraviolet (UV) light, mutagenesis of the DNA in somatic cells is no different from that in the germline. Some is **spontaneous**, caused by a base adopting a variant molecular form or **tautomer** during DNA replication; most is initiated by chemicals and 10–15% by radiation. For the natural mutation rate, see Chapter 17.

## Chemical mutagenesis

Environmental **mutagens** include constituents of smoke, paints, petrochemicals, pesticides, dyes, foodstuffs, drugs, etc. Examples of the major categories are given below. The principal means of exposure are inhalation, skin absorption and ingestion. **Promutagens**, such as *nitrates* and *nitrites* are converted into mutagens by body chemistry.

**1 Base analogues**. *2-amino-purine* is incorporated into DNA in place of adenine, but pairs as cytosine, causing a **substitution** of thymine by guanine in the partner strand. *5-bromouracil* (5-BU) is incorporated as thymine, but can undergo a tautomeric shift to resemble cytosine, resulting in a **transition** from T-A to C-G.

**2 Chemical modifiers**. *Nitrous acid* converts cytosine to uracil, and adenine to hypoxanthine, a precursor of guanine. *Alkylating agents* modify bases by donating alkyl groups.

**3 Intercalating agents**. The antiseptic *proflavine* and the *acridine dyes* become inserted between adjacent base pairs, producing distortions in the DNA that lead to **deletions** and **additions**.

**4 Other**. A wide range of other chemicals cause DNA **strand breakage** and **cross-linking**.

## Electromagnetic radiation

Particulate discharge from radioactive decay includes alpha-particles (helium nuclei), beta-particles (electrons) and gamma-rays. The mutagenicity of subatomic particles depends on their speed, mass and electric charge.

The mutagenicity of electromagnetic radiation increases with decreasing wavelength. All radiation beyond UV causes ionization by knocking electrons out of their orbits.

### UV light

UV light is the non-visible, short wavelength fraction of sunlight. It exerts a mutagenic effect by causing **dimerization** (linking) of adjacent pyrimidine residues, mainly T-T (but also T-C and C-C). It does not cause germline mutations, but is a major cause of skin cancer, especially in homozygotes for the red hair allele (see Chapter 16), who have white, freckled skin.

Most UV radiation from the sun is blocked by a 4-mm layer of ozone in the upper atmosphere, but this is currently under destruction by industrial *fluorocarbons*.

### Atomic radiation

**1 Natural background radiation**. This varies with local geology. The most abundant radioisotopes are Potassium-40 and Radon-222 gas. Radon contributes 55% of all natural background radiation and may be responsible for 2500 deaths per annum in the UK.

**2 Cosmic rays**. These present a major theoretical hazard for aircrews, as their intensity increases with altitude. Exposure during a return flight between England and Spain may equal five chest X-rays.

**3 Man-made radiation**. This includes fallout from nuclear testing and power stations. Radiation workers are at particular risk and bone-surface-seeking isotopes present a major risk of leukaemia.

**4 X-rays**. X-rays account for 60% of man-made and 11% of total radiation exposure. They mutagenize DNA either directly by ionizing impact, or indirectly by creating highly reactive **free radicals** that impinge on the DNA. These can be carried in the bloodstream and harm cells not directly exposed.

## Biological effects of radiation

Electomagnetic radiation damages proteins and above 100 rads kills cells. (One **rad** is the amount of radiation that causes one gram of tissue to absorb 100 ergs of energy.) At the chromosomal level it causes **major deletions**, **translocations** and **aneuploidy** (see Table 47.1). It causes **single-** and **double-strand breaks** in DNA and **base pair destruction**. X-rays damage chromosomes most readily when they are condensed, which is why they are most harmful to dividing cells, including the progenitors of sperm. The offspring of older men have a many-fold risk of genetic disease, as the DNA in their sperm has been copied many times (see figure). The high testicular temperature caused by clothing (6°C above unclothed) has been estimated to be responsible for half the present mutation rate in human sperm.

For the first 7 days of life the embryo is ultra-sensitive to the mutagenic and lethal effects of X-rays; over weeks 2–7 teratogenic effects come to the fore. Childhood leukaemia can be induced by exposure at gestational weeks 8–40.

At 100 rads X-rays cause a 50% reduction in white blood cell count, while whole-body irradiation of 450 rads kills 50% of people. Therapeutic doses of up to 1000 rads are used against cancer cells. Radiation damage is cumulative and there is no lower baseline of effect.

## Safety measures when using X-rays

**1** *Patients' previous X-ray exposure should be reviewed before requesting further X-rays.*

**2** *The '28-day Rule': a woman of child-bearing age should be X-rayed only if she has had a period within the last 28 days.*

**3** *Patients with DNA repair deficiencies should NEVER be X-rayed.*

## DNA repair

Apart from direct repair, all the DNA repair systems in human cells require **exonucleases**, **endonucleases** (defective in **Cocayne syndrome**), **polymerases** and **ligases**. **Ataxia telangiectasia** and **Fanconi anaemia** patients have defects in DNA damage detection and are extremely sensitive to X-rays.

**1 Direct repair**. A specific enzyme reverses the damage, e.g. by de-alkylation of alkylated guanine.

**2 Base-excision repair**. The damaged base, plus a few others on either side, are removed by cutting the sugar-phosphate backbone and the gap filled by re-synthesis directed by the intact strand.

**3 Nucleotide excision repair**. This removes **thymine dimers** and chemically modified bases over a longer stretch of DNA. Defects can cause **xeroderma pigmentosum**.

**4 Mismatch repair**. This corrects base mismatches due to errors at DNA replication and involves nicking the faulty strand at the nearest GATC base sequence. Defects occur in **hereditary non-polyposis colon cancer**.

**5 Postreplication repair**. This corrects double-strand breaks either unguided, or by using the homologous chromosome as a template. Defects occur in **Bloom syndrome** (a '**chromosome breakage syndrome**') and **breast cancer**.

## Types of mutation

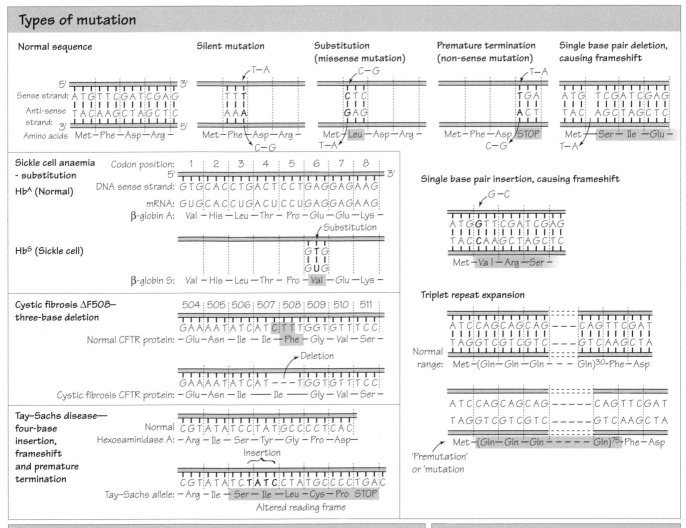

**Sickle cell anaemia - substitution**

**Cystic fibrosis ΔF508– three-base deletion**

**Tay–Sachs disease— four-base insertion, frameshift and premature termination**

## Causation of red and green colour vision anomalies (in males) due to unequal crossing-over (in females) between the X-linked red and green photosensitive pigment genes

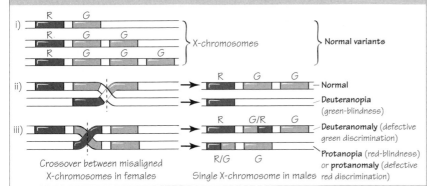

## Table 30.1 Diseases caused by triplet repeats

| Disease | Triplet | Location | Inheritance |
|---|---|---|---|
| Huntington disease | CAG | Exon | Aut. dom. |
| Myotonic dystrophy | CTG | 3' UTR | Aut. dom. |
| Fragile X (Frax-A) | CGG | 5' UTR | X-l. rec. |
| Frax-E | CCG | Promoter | X-linked |
| Frax-F | GCC | ? | X-linked |
| Spino-cerebellar ataxias (SCA 1, 2, 3, 6, 7) | CAG | Exon | Aut. dom. |
| SCA 8 | CTG | UTR | Autosomal |
| Spino-bulbar muscular atrophy (Kennedy disease) | CAG | Exon | X-l. rec. |
| Friedrich ataxia | GAA | Intron | Aut. rec. |
| Dentatorubral-pallidoluysian atrophy (DRPLA) | CAG | Exon | Aut. dom. |

UTR, untranslated region

## Overview

**Mutations** are permanent modifications of DNA. They include aneuploidies (see Chapter 14), chromosome rearrangements (see Chapter 15), **point mutations**, involving **substitution**, **deletion** or **insertion** of a base pair, DNA **duplications** and **inversions** and **RNA processing mutations**.

Large deletions and insertions can be created by **unequal crossing over** between misaligned segments of repetitious DNA causing, for example, anomalous colour vision (see figure).

**Dynamic mutations** are progressive and involve expansion of **triplet repeat sequences**.

## Substitutions, deletions, insertions and frameshifts

Substitution involves replacement of a base pair. If the amino acid coded by the new codon is the same, it is a **silent mutation**, or if different, a **missense mutation**. Most missense mutations are harmful, but a notable exception is the substitution of the sixth codon in the β-globin chain responsible for sickle cell anaemia (see Chapter 25), which in heterozygotes confers resistance to *falciparum* malaria.

Substitution can create a STOP codon, causing translation to come to a premature halt. This is called a **premature termination** or **non-sense mutation**.

If a deleted or inserted segment is of other than a multiple of three bases, apart from loss or gain of coding information, the translation reading frame is disrupted in a **frameshift mutation**. This causes the protein produced to be entirely erroneous 'downstream' (3′) of the deletion. The most common mutation causing **Tay–Sachs disease** (see Chapter 18) is a four-base insertion causing a frameshift and leading to premature termination, so that no functional **hexosaminidase A** is synthesized.

### Transcriptional control

Mutations in the flanking regions of genes can have quantitative effects by inhibiting binding of transcription factors, as in the **Factor IX** gene 5′ region, causing **haemophilia B**.

### RNA processing

**Splicing mutants** either directly affect hnRNA donor or acceptor sites (see Chapter 7), or activate cryptic competitive splice sites in introns or exons. The acceptor sequence at the end of the first intron of β-globin is UUAGGCU, while within that intron is a sequence that differs by two bases: UUGGUCU. In some beta-thalassaemia patients the latter is modified to UUAGUCU. Since this differs by only one base from the normal acceptor it gets misidentified as the acceptor, the hnRNA is cut in the wrong place and the resultant mRNA erroneously retains some intron bases. This in turn introduces a frameshift, causing 'CUU AGG' to be read as '-CU UAG G-'. Translation ceases prematurely because UAG is a STOP signal, resulting in **β⁺-thalassaemia** (see below).

In one RNA processing mutation an A-to-C transition of the first nucleotide of the β-globin messenger inhibits capping, while in another, substitution of U by C in the trailer sequence AAUAAA inhibits polyadenylation (see Chapter 7). Both fail to suppress rapid degradation of the messenger.

## Thalassaemia

The thalassaemias are collectively the most common single gene disorder, in all of which there is reduced level of synthesis of either the α-, or β-globin chain (see Chapter 25). In the absence of a complementary chain with which to form the haemoglobin tetramer (α2β2), the chain produced at the normal rate is in relative excess and precipitates out, damaging the red cell membranes and leading to their premature destruction.

### Beta-thalassaemia

There are at least 80 beta-thalassaemia alleles in addition to the RNA splicing error above (see Table 25.2). Most of these are point mutations and most patients are 'compound homozygotes', with two *different* deficient alleles. Carriers of one beta-thalassaemia allele have slight anaemia and are said to have **β⁺-thalassaemia**, or **thalassaemia minor**. If no β-globin is present, the condition is **β⁰-thalassaemia**, or **thalassaemia major**.

In **hereditary persistence of fetal haemoglobin**, the β-globin gene has been deleted and the neighbouring γ-globin gene responsible for **fetal haemoglobin** (α2γ2), remains transcriptionally active at a high level after birth.

### Alpha-thalassaemia

Alpha-globin is coded by *two pairs* of genes per diploid genome. In the 'heterozygous' state, called **alpha-thalassaemia trait**, there are two mutant and two normal genes, either −α/−α, or −/αα (see Table 25.1). The latter is relatively common in South-East Asia and gives rise to completely α-globin deficient homozygotes (--/--) with **hydrops foetalis**. The (−α) haplotype is unusually common (αα) among Melanesians, having been selected by malaria (see Chapter 25).

In **Haemoglobin Constant Spring** the UAA α-globin STOP codon is mutated to CAA, coding for glutamine, and translation continues for a further 31 frames to another STOP. The mutant mRNA is unstable, causing mild alpha-thalassaemia.

## Dynamic mutation: triplet repeat disorders

Modification of the genetic material can occur by expansion or contraction of **trinucleotide**, or **triplet repeats**. There are close to 20 diseases in this category and most show dominant inheritance (Table 30.1).

**1 Myotonic dystrophy** involves repeats of **CTG** in the 3′ (downstream) regulatory region.

**2 Huntington disease** has extra repeats of **CAG** in an exon, that create a run of glutamines in the protein. The normal range is 6 to ~35 repeats, patients have 37–121.

**3 Fragile X disease** (**Frax-A**) involves repeats of **CGG** in the 5′ (upstream) region, two to 60 copies being the norm. Sixty to 200 copies represent a **premutation** which can expand further in offspring. At over 200 repeats the gene becomes methylated and fails to produce the protein **FMR-1**, causing mental retardation and other disease symptoms.

*As triplet repeat series expand from one generation to the next, disease symptoms become more severe and appear at progressively younger ages.* This is called **anticipation**. In myotonic dystrophy and Fragile X disease, expansion occurs in the mother; in Huntington disease expansion occurs in the father.

## Nomenclature of mutations

Mutations are named by conventional abbreviations. For example, the most common mutation responsible for cystic fibrosis is **ΔF508**. The symbol 'Δ' denotes a deletion, F stands for phenylalanine and 508 indicates the location of the mutation in the coding sequence of the gene for the 'cystic fibrosis trans-membrane regulator' (**CFTR**).

## The signal transduction cascade

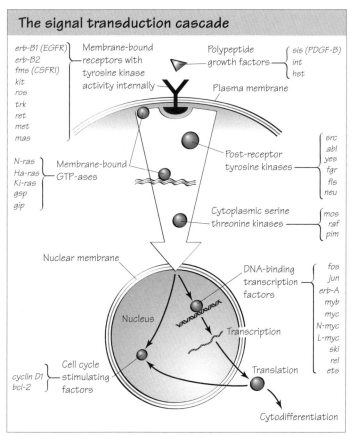

## Hereditary and sporadic retinoblastoma; the basis of the two-hit hypothesis

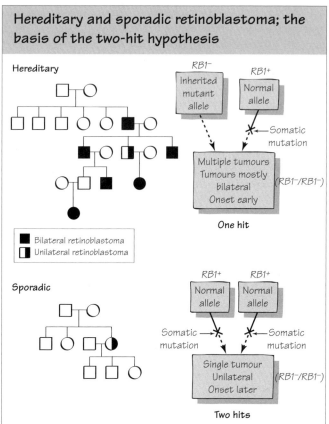

## Molecular events during development of familial adenomatous polyposis (*FAP*); the basis of the multi-hit hypothesis

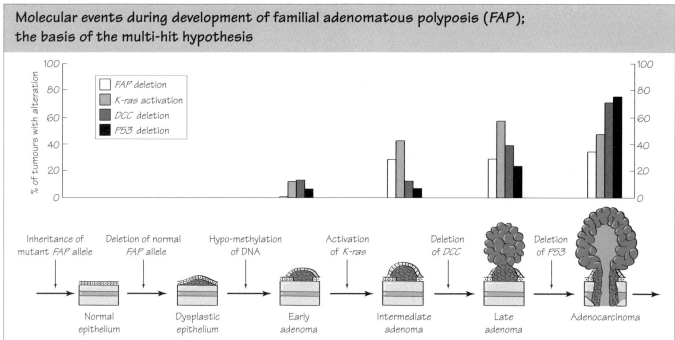

## Overview

Normal progress through the cell cycle is promoted by polypeptide **growth factors** that bind to specific receptors on the cell surface. Their presence is conveyed to the nucleus by a series of phosphorylations of **kinases** (phosphate-attaching enzymes) that constitute the **signal transduction cascade (STC)**. Phosphorylated **DNA binding proteins** then bind to specific sites in the DNA and promote transition to the next phase of the cycle. The genes that code for the (normal) proteins involved in the STC are **proto-oncogenes**. Cancer-causing derivatives are called **oncogenes**.

Progress through the cycle is moderated by the protein products of the **mitosis suppressor** (or '**tumour suppressor**') **genes** (see Chapter 9) and cancers are frequently initiated by their failure. The properties of tumour suppressor genes and oncogenes are compared in Table 32.1.

Cancer cells can invade neighbouring tissues or undergo **metastasis**, i.e. break up and move in the blood to establish **secondary tumours** in distant parts of the body.

If a tumour shows sustained proliferation and spread it is said to be 'malignant', being capable of causing death, most often by pressure or occlusion. Malignant cells typically lack **contact inhibition of movement**, **density dependent inhibition of growth** and the normal requirement of a rigid substratum for mitosis, allowing them to invade and proliferate to abnormal extent. 'Benign' tumours usually do not spread, either by local invasion or metastasis.

## Environmental triggers

Most mutagens (see Chapter 29) can trigger **carcinogenesis**. Non-mutagenic cancer-promoting chemicals operate by activation of kinases.

## Viruses

Viruses can '**transform**' normal cells into cancer cells by insertion of a viral promoter beside a host proto-oncogene (as with **Epstein–Barr virus** in some cases of Burkitt lymphoma), or by introduction of a viral genome that already carries an oncogene. Some of the latter are replication-competent **transforming viruses**, but in most cases an additional '**helper virus**' is needed for replication.

DNA viruses implicated in human cancer include **papilloma**, Epstein–Barr and **hepatitis B**. Oncogenic RNA retroviruses include **T cell leukaemia virus** and **Kaposi sarcoma associated herpes virus**.

## The signal transduction cascade

**1 Growth factors.** Growth factors promote transition of cells from G0 to G1 (see Chapter 9). The best-known is *c-sis*, identical to the B subunit of **platelet derived growth factor**. Two others, *hst* and *int-2*, have been found amplified in stomach cancers and malignant melanomas, respectively.

**2 Growth factor receptors.** Growth factor receptors span the cell membrane and have tyrosine kinase properties at their cytoplasmic ends. An example is *c-erb-B*, which encodes **epidermal growth factor receptor**. Activation of *erb-B2* independently of growth factor stimulation is associated with cancer of the stomach, pancreas and ovary.

**3 Postreceptor tyrosine kinases.** The target of kinase activity of the growth factor receptor is characteristically a **postreceptor tyrosine kinase**, which in turn phosphorylates another cytoplasmic kinase that phosphorylates a third, and so on.

**4 Serine threonine kinases.** Some steps in the STC involve phosphorylation of serine or threonine residues by, for example, the *raf* protein. Mutant versions of *raf* maintain continuous transmission of the growth-promoting signal.

**5 GTPases.** Phosphate for kinase activity is largely supplied by ATP, but the intracellular membranes carry GTPases also, including three *ras* proteins. Mutations resulting in increased or sustained GTPase activity lead to continuous growth.

**6 DNA binding proteins and cell cycle factors.** DNA-binding onco-proteins control expression of genes concerned with the cell cycle. Over-production of *myc* and *myb*, which stimulate transition from G1 to S-phase, prevents cells from entering G0.

Loss of factors that normally cause **apoptosis** (cell death) results in tumour build up and activation of *bcl-2*, through chromosome rearrangement, inhibiting apoptosis in some lymphomas.

## Conversion of proto-oncogenes to oncogenes

**1 Point mutation.** Thirty per cent of tumours contain mutated versions of one or other of the *ras* proteins that are unable to adopt the inactive form.

**2 Translocation.** Examples are the Philadelphia chromosome (see Chapter 32) and translocations of *myc* on Chromosome 8, to alongside the promoters of the Ig heavy chain on Chromosome 14, the kappa light chain on Chromosome 2, or the lambda light chain on 22 (see Chapter 33). These are found in at least 90% of cases of Burkitt lymphoma.

**3 Insertional mutagenesis.** See 'Viruses' above.

**4 Amplification.** In 10% of tumours are tiny, supernumerary pieces of DNA called **double-minute chromosomes** composed of amplified copies of a proto-oncogene, e.g. of *N-myc* in some neuroblastomas and *erb-B2* in breast cancers. Amplified proto-oncogenes inserted into chromosomes are detectable as **homogeneously staining regions**, or **HSRs**.

## P53: 'the guardian of the genome'

Point mutations and deletions of P53 occur in 70% of all tumours. Its protein acts as a tumour suppressor, contributing to the G1 block and so allowing time for DNA defects to be detected and repaired. P53 also mediates commitment to apoptosis.

Li–Fraumeni syndrome, due to a germline defect in P53, is notable for its assortment of tumours (see Chapter 32).

## The two-hit hypothesis

Retinoblastoma, can be: (a) sporadic, unilateral, with average age of onset 30 months, or (b) familial, bilateral, with average age of onset 14 months and accompanied by other cancers.

The normal allele for retinoblastoma (RB1$^{1+}$) is a tumour suppressor that blocks mitosis of retinal cells at the G1/S transition. Knudson's **two-hit hypothesis** proposed that cancer develops only if *both* RB alleles are inactive. In familial cases one lesion is inherited. Only one further mutation *in any retinal cell* is necessary, so it occurs much earlier than in normal homozygotes (see figure).

## The multi-hit hypothesis
### Cancer of the colon

In **familial adenomatous polyposis (coli) (FAP(C))** inheritance of a single mutant tumour suppressor allele is associated with multiple benign polyps (**adenomas**) of the colon lining. Progression toward an **adenocarcinoma** begins with deletion of the normal allele. Subsequent steps involve activation of the *K-ras* oncogene and deletion of P53. Deletion of the '**Deleted in Colorectal Carcinoma**' (**DCC**) gene initiates cell surface changes and further mutation promotes metastasis and early death. The specific mutations described are characteristic, but can occur in any order (see figure).

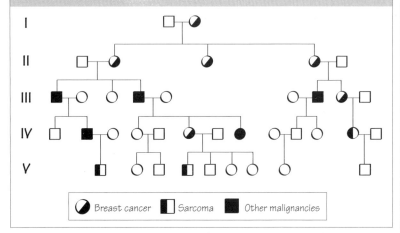

A pedigree for Li–Fraumeni syndrome showing breast cancer, sarcomas and other malignancies, with general susceptibility to cancer inherited in a dominant fashion. (From Li, F. P. (1998) *Cancer Research* 48; 5381–6)

Breast cancer | Sarcoma | Other malignancies

## Table 32.1 Comparison of the properties of oncogenes and tumour suppressor genes

| Oncogenes | Tumour suppressor genes |
|---|---|
| (Over-) active in tumour | Normal allele inactive in tumour |
| (Over-) activity associated with translocation or substitution | Abnormality due to deletion or specific mutation of normal allele |
| Abnormality rarely inherited | Abnormality can be inherited |
| Dominant at cellular level | Recessive at cellular level |
| Broad tissue specificity | Considerable tumour specificity |
| Frequently causative of leukaemia and lymphoma | Causative of solid tumours |

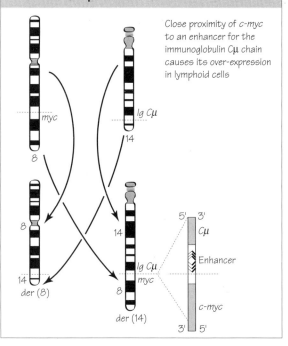

### Typical 8:14 translocation causing Burkitt lymphoma

Close proximity of *c-myc* to an enhancer for the immunoglobulin Cμ chain causes its over-expression in lymphoid cells

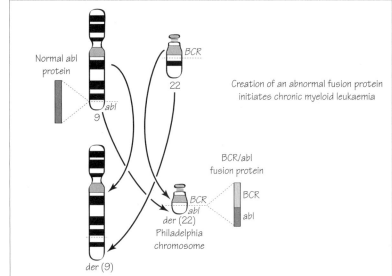

### Derivation of the Philadelphia chromosome by reciprocal exchange between chromosomes 9 and 22

Creation of an abnormal fusion protein initiates chronic myeloid leukaemia

## Overview

All cancer is genetic at the level of the cell. **Oncogenesis**, i.e. cancer development, is a multistage process during which a cell accumulates damage in several critical genes related to mitosis, such as the proto-oncogenes (Chapter 31). A small proportion develop as a consequence of genetic predisposition that includes pale (e.g. Northern European) skin pigmentation, red hair with associated freckling (Chapter 16) and defective DNA repair genes (Chapter 29). Dominant inheri-

tance patterns are generally due to a defective tumour suppressor gene (coding for a mitosis suppressor protein; Chapter 9 and Table 32.1).

## Indicators of inherited cancer

Familial clusters can be caused by shared environments; the following are pointers to genetic causation.
1 Several close relatives with the same, or genetically associated cancers.

**2** Two family members with the same rare cancer.

**3** Unusually early age of onset.

**4** Bilateral tumours in paired organs.

**5** Non-clonal multifocal or successive tumours in the same tissue, or in different organ systems of the same individual.

## Recessive DNA repair defects
### Damage detection errors

**1 Ataxia telangiectasia**—autosomal recessive (AR); frequency: 1/50 000. There is hypersensitivity to X-rays, rearrangement of Chromosomes 7 and 14, cerebellar degeneration and enlargement of capillaries (**telangiectasis**) in the cornea. A 35% risk of lymphoreticular malignancy leads to early death in 30% of cases.

**2 Fanconi anaemia**—AR; frequency: 1/350 000. There is undue sensitivity to DNA cross-linking agents, with chromosome breakage, and a 5–10% risk of leukaemia and carcinomas.

### Nucleotide excision repair defects

**Xeroderma pigmentosum (XP)**—AR, at least 7 types; frequency 1/250 000. Errors in pyrimidine dimer excision lead to multiple skin cancers, with corneal scarring and early death.

### Post-replication repair errors

**Bloom syndrome**—AR. There is a 10-fold rate of sister chromatid exchange, typically causing short stature and increased risk of leukaemia, lymphoma and carcinoma.

## Tumour suppressor genes
### Dominant DNA repair defects
*DNA mismatch repair*

**Hereditary non-polyposis colon cancer**—autosomal dominant (AD). Several known defects in GATC endonuclease (Chapter 29) cause early onset colon and endometrial cancer.

*Post-replication repair*

**Familial breast cancer, BRCA1, BRCA2**—(AD); frequency: ~1/200. One in eight British women develop breast and/or ovarian cancer, about 5% of these having inherited susceptibility. BRCA1 and BRCA2 account for well over half of these. The age-related penetrance for ovarian cancer is 40–60% for BRCA1, 10–20% for BRCA2.

### Cell cycle block defects

**1 Familial retinoblastoma**—AD with 90% penetrance; frequency: 1/18 000 (see Chapter 31).

**2 Li–Fraumeni syndrome**—AD. This is due to an inherited defect in P53; see figure and Chapter 31.

### Intracellular signal defects

**1 Neurofibromatosis Type 1 (NF1; von Recklinghausen disease)**—AD; frequency: 1/3000. Loss of the NF1 normal protein allows accumulation of **ras-GTP**, with increased cell turnover (see Chapter 31). There are numerous prominent benign fibromas and malignant tumours of the central nervous system.

**2 Neurofibromatosis Type 2 (NF2)**—AD; frequency: 1/35 000. There are bilateral Schwann cell fibromas of auditory and spinal nerves and intracranial meningiomas.

**3 Familial adenomatous polyposis (FAP)** Types 1 and 3—AD; combined frequency: 1/10 000. There are multiple benign polyps of the colon, with 90% risk of malignancy and **retinal hypertrophy** in 80% of families (see Chapter 31).

### Transcriptional control defects

**1 Von Hippel–Lindau syndrome**—AD; frequency: 1/36 000. There are **haemangioblastomas** of the retina and cerebellum, early onset renal carcinomas and **phaeochromocytomas**, especially of the adrenal gland.

**2 Wilms' tumour (nephroblastoma)**—AD; frequency: 1/10 000. This is a highly malignant kidney tumour; 1% of cases is familial. It forms part of the **contiguous gene syndrome WAGR** (**W**ilms tumour, **A**niridia, **G**enitourinary anomalies and mental **R**etardation) caused by a major deletion.

### Cytodifferentiative errors

**Basal cell naevus (Gorlin) syndrome**—AD; frequency: 1/57 000. There are skin naevi from puberty and a predisposition to basal cell carcinoma, medulloblastoma and ovarian fibromas. There are also dental malformations, cleft palate and bifid ribs. Patients are unduly sensitive to radiation.

## Oncogenes
### Growth factor reception

**Multiple endocrine neoplasia, Type 2 (MEN 2).** This is an autosomal dominant syndrome of multiple endocrine neoplasms, including medullary thyroid carcinoma, phaeochromocytoma and parathyroid adenomas. There is gain of function of **c-ret**.

### Signal transduction

**Chronic myeloid (or myelogenous) leukaemia (CML).** Translocation of *c-abl*, normally on 9q, to a position beside the '**breakpoint cluster region**' (*BCR*) on 22q initiates synthesis of a chimaeric '**fusion protein**' with increased tyrosine kinase activity. Reciprocal exchange of the 22 telomere leaves a characteristic modified version of 22, the '**Philadelphia chromosome**', in the affected cell line.

### DNA binding

**Burkitt lymphoma.** This is a B-lymphocyte tumour of the jaw, the most common childhood cancer of equatorial Africa. The proto-oncogene *c-myc* at 8q24 becomes activated by translocation adjacent to an immunoglobulin enhancer at 14q32, 2p11 or 22q11.

# 33 Immunogenetics

## The major histocompatibility complex

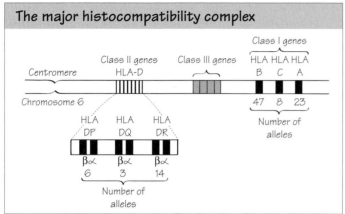

## A secreted immunoglobulin molecule

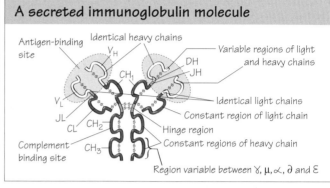

## Genetic events leading to synthesis of an immunoglobulin kappa light chain

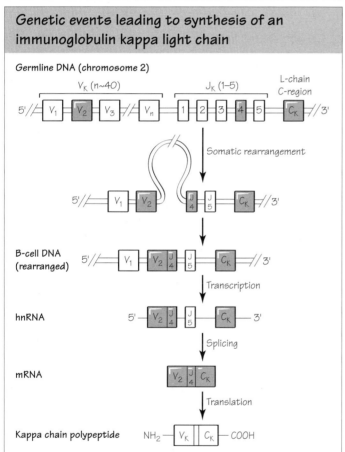

## Class I MHC molecule (HLA-A, -B, -C)

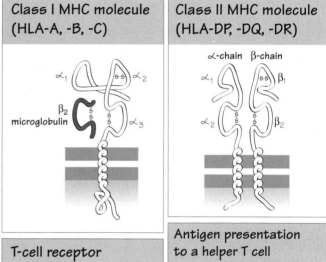

## Class II MHC molecule (HLA-DP, -DQ, -DR)

## T-cell receptor

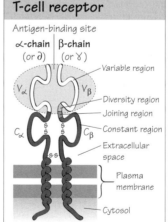

## Antigen presentation to a helper T cell

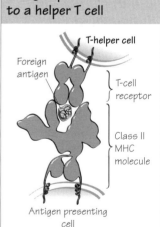

## Overview

Immunogenetics concerns the genetics of the **immune system**, the exceptionally sensitive system that defends the body against invading pathogens and rejects malignant cells or incompatible tissue grafts. The relevance of the ABO and Rhesus blood group systems to transplantation is discussed in Chapter 25.

In a simplified description, three classes of cells are involved, all derived from bone-marrow stem cells. One population migrates to the spleen and lymph nodes and becomes **B-lymphocytes**, which secrete an infinite variety of soluble **immunoglobulins**, or **antibodies**.

The second population migrates to the thymus and develops into **T-lymphocytes**. These differentiate into **T4 cells** (**helpers** and **induc-**

ers), **T8 cells** (**cytotoxic** and **suppressor cells**) and **natural killer cells**. T-cells carry an infinite variety of antigen receptors.

**Macrophages** are the third class. They move directly into the circulation.

The **humoral immune response** is initiated by macrophages. For example, they engulf virally infected cells and pass viral antigens to the T4 helper cells. These activate immature B-cells and T8 suppressor cells. The B-cells then proliferate and differentiate into **plasma cells** that secrete antibodies which destroy the virus. The T8 suppressors later suppress B-cell activity.

The **cellular immune response** is initiated by T4 inducer cells, upon contact with foreign antigen. They trigger maturation of immature T-cells, causing their differentiation into cytotoxic T8 cells capable of destroying invading pathogens. Natural killer cells attack pathogens and destroy antigens *without* mediation by helper cells.

Specification for specific responses is retained by **memory B-** and **T-cells**.

Three kinds of molecules important in these interactions are the **MHC proteins**, the **immunoglobulins** and the **T-cell receptors** (**TCRs**).

## The major histocompatibilty complex

MHC proteins are present on the surfaces of all nucleated cells. **They show wide polymorphism** (see Chapter 25), **but are uniform within an individual**. *In the context of transplantation* they act as antigens.

The Class I MHC proteins consist of a heavy chain encoded by gene HLA-A, HLA-B or HLA-C, which links with a molecule of **β2-microglobulin**. Class II (HLA-D) proteins are heterodimers of alpha and beta sub-units and are present only on B lymphocytes. Both Class I and Class II antigens play critical roles in the 'presentation' of foreign antigens to T lymphocytes.

The Class III genes encode components of the **complement** system, concerned with cell lysis.

## The immunoglobulins

Within each person a different species of immunoglobulin is produced for every potential foreign antigen. *This enormous diversity is created by unique kinds of genetic rearrangement within individual B-lymphocytes* (see figure).

An immunoglobulin (Ig) molecule has two **heavy** (H) chains and a pair of **kappa** (κ) or **lambda** (λ) **light** (L) chains. The latter consist of **constant** (C), **variable** (V) and **joining** (J) **regions**.

There are of five classes of heavy chain defined by their C-regions: **IgG**, **IgM**, **IgA**, **IgD** and **IgE**, with heavy chains **gamma** (γ); **mu** (μ); **alpha** (α); **delta** (δ) and **epsilon** (ε), respectively. There is also a '**hinge**' and V, J and **diversity** (D) **regions**.

There are around 40 alternative sequences within the kappa L-chain V region, five in the J, and one C gene, on Chromosome 2. The lambda genes on Chromosome 22 show similar complexity. For the heavy chains, there are nine C genes (γ, μ, etc., on Chromosome 14), plus about 20 D between the arrays of V and J genes. *The different B-cells of one individual synthesize billions of different specificities of antibody by differential splicing of these alternative sequences, their transcripts*

*being edited further at the RNA stage. Different pairs of H and L chains then link as symmetrical tetramers.*

*Within one B-cell antigen-binding specificity can be transferred between different heavy chains.* When a B-cell produces both IgG and IgM, of the same specificity it acquires competence to respond to antigen and, on contact with that antigen, proliferates and produces antibody in profusion.

## The T-cell receptor

The TCRs play key roles in antigen recognition and helper activity, but a T-cell responds to a foreign antigen only if it is complexed with an MHC molecule.

The TCRs are dimers composed usually of a TCR α and β chain (or else a TCR γ and δ chain). *Their genes also have separate segments that are alternatively spliced to create extensive diversity.*

## Genetic disorders of the immune system
### Absence of B-cell (humoral) immunity
**X-linked agammaglobulinaemia.** This is rare and usually affects only boys, when, at 5–6 months, they become highly susceptible to bacterial infection. It is characterized by a defect in a **protein kinase**, affecting maturation of B-cells.

### Absence of T-cell (cellular) immunity
**1  T-cell immunodeficiency, or nucleoside phosphorylase deficiency**—AR. This causes a gradual decline in T lymphocytes, leading to recurring viral and fungal infections from 3 months after birth.
**2  DiGeorge syndrome.** This is due to deletion of several contiguous genes at 22q11, causing absence of the thymus.
**3  Chediak–Higashi syndrome**—AR. Only the natural killer cells are affected. One of its features is malignant lymphoma.

### Total absence of both B-cell and T-cell immunity
**Severe combined immunodeficiency syndrome (SCID).** There are X-linked and autosomal recessive forms. About half of the latter involve deficiency of **adenosine deaminase** (**ADA**; see also Chapter 48).

### Autoimmune disease
Soon after birth the immune system develops tolerance to all the body's accessible antigens. In autoimmune disease, tolerance breaks down, triggered usually by injury or infection. Cytotoxic T-cells then proliferate and attack the patient's own tissues.

Autoimmune diseases may be **organ-specific**, e.g. **Hashimoto thyroiditis**; or **systemic**, e.g. **systemic lupus erythematosus**. Autoimmune diseases are most common in women and typically show association with specific HLA alleles (see Chapter 27). Explanations for this include:
**1** close genetic linkage of disease susceptibility genes to the HLA complex and survival of the original haplotypes (linkage disequilibrium);
**2** cross-reactivity between specific HLA antigens and antibodies to specific environmental antigens;
**3** incomplete or erroneous development of tolerance.

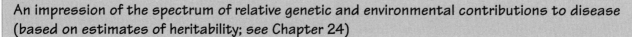

An impression of the spectrum of relative genetic and environmental contributions to disease (based on estimates of heritability; see Chapter 24)

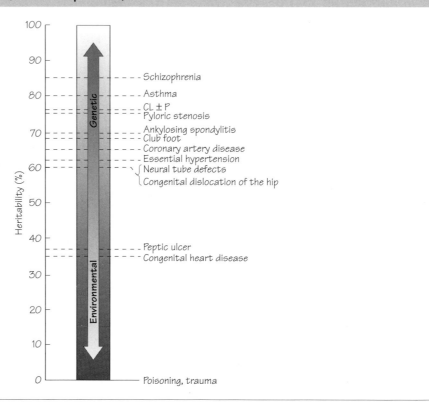

## Overview

Genetics underpins and potentially overlaps all other clinical topics, but is especially relevant to reproduction, paediatrics, epidemiology, therapeutics and nursing. It offers unprecedented opportunities for prevention and avoidance of disease because genetic disorders can often be predicted long before the onset of symptoms. This is known as **predictive** or **presymptomatic genetics**. Currently healthy populations can be screened for persons with a particular genotype that might cause later trouble for them or their children.

Genetic advice to patients and their families should be **non-directive, non-judgemental** and **supportive**, and can be summarized by four words: **communication, comprehension, care** and **confidentiality**.

## Communication

For the genetic counsellor and the health visitor good communication skills are vital, as what they convey to a family can have profound implications not only for their present happiness, but for the health of that family for ever more. When assembling information they should preserve a warm and non-judgemental attitude, take adequate time and remember to consider their own body language. It is common for people to experience fear, denial, anger or guilt, but reassurance from an authoritative figure outside the family can help them come to terms with such feelings.

Family myths often grow up around genetic disorders and these must be explored and disentangled before concepts such as X-linked, dominant or recessive inheritance will be accepted. Family secrets such as incestuous or extra-marital relationships may be revealed during the investigation and may be critical to the assessment of genetic risk. Such problem areas must be treated with extreme discretion.

Following face-to-face consultation it is usual to write to the family to reiterate the main points and re-address difficult aspects.

## Comprehension

An important principle is that *where possible, diagnosis should precede counselling*, but in some cases supportive counselling is needed before a definitive diagnosis has been achieved. Examples include unknown dysmorphic syndromes, children with dysmorphic features who are too young to have 'grown into' a recognizable syndrome and conditions in which there is marked genetic heterogeneity.

Initial contact with the consultand usually involves construction of a 'family tree' or **pedigree diagram** (see Chapter 35). Physical examination for dysmorphic features can play a significant part in genetic diagnosis and guidance on this is given in Chapter 37.

Looking at chromosomes provides a broad overview of the genome (see Chapter 38), in contrast to the molecular genetics approach where tests are for one or a few specific mutations (see Chapters 42–45). The assessment of risks can be exceedingly complex, but instructive examples are given in Chapter 36. DNA fingerprinting, as described in Chapter 46, is of enormous value in paternity testing and other forensic aspects of medicine.

The genetic counsellor will generally have been trained in psychology as well as general medicine, clinical genetics and possibly other medical disciplines, but his or her comprehension is further informed by a team of experts. This generally includes additional medically trained clinical geneticists, laboratory scientists including cytogeneticists and molecular biologists, and genetic nurses.

## Care

After taking family details and constructing a family tree it is necessary

**Table 34.1** Genetic isolates with high frequency of certain autosomal disorders.

| Population | Disease |
| --- | --- |
| Old-order Amish (Pennsylvania) | Chondroectodermal dysplasia<br>Ellis–van Creveld syndrome<br>Cartilage–hair hypoplasia |
| Kuna (San Blas) Indians (Panama) | Albinism |
| Hopi Indians (Arizona) | Albinism |
| Pima Indians (US South-west) | Non-insulin dependent diabetes mellitus |
| Finns | Congenital chloride diarrhoea<br>Aspartylglycosaminuria<br>Congenital nephrotic syndrome<br>MULIBREY–nanism |
| Yupik Eskimo | Congenital adrenal hyperplasia |
| Afrikaaners (South Africa) | Porphyria variegata<br>Familial hypercholesterolaemia<br>Lipoid proteinosis<br>Huntington disease<br>Sclereosteosis |
| Ashkenzi Jews | Tay–Sachs disease<br>Gaucher disease<br>Dysautonomia<br>Canavan disease |
| Karaite Jews | Werdnig–Hoffmann disease |
| Ryukyan Islands (Japan) | Spinal muscular atrophy |
| Cypriots, Sardinians | Beta-thalassaemia |

to assess what the consultand actually wants to know: there may be specific concerns that are not obvious to the counsellor. Individuals should, when possible, be offered the choice of more than one alternative; for example, between presymptomatic testing and medical surveillance alone. The concept of 'high risk' is subjective, but comparison of genetic risks with statistics on other aspects of health can help put things in perspective (see Table 40.2).

Genetically based disease varies between ethnic groups (Table 34.1) and some knowledge of the family's educational, social and religious backgrounds is also important as these affect their reactions and decision-making. Consultation can create new uncertainties and individuals may adopt a coping style known as 'functional pessimism' to protect themselves from future disappointments. Guilt and depression can arise in those who receive favourable test results when their relatives are less fortunate. Long-term emotional support should therefore be offered at the same time as any offer of predictive testing.

Population screening for disease alleles, combined with appropriate courses of action has yielded dramatic reductions in disease incidence (see Chapter 47). However, 'eugenic' concepts that conceive genetic improvement at the *population* level and issues such as cost-saving or contribution to research should not influence decisions made by individuals regarding their own lives or those of their offspring. Potential ethical problems are minimized if the *rights of individuals* are given priority.

It should be remembered that diagnosis of high liability toward genetic disease is not necessarily an irrevocable condemnation to ill health. As stressed in Chapter 1, phenotypic characters are the product of interaction between genotype and environment acting over time; in some cases optimal health can be maintained only by avoidance of genotype-specific environmental hazards (see Chapters 47 and 48).

## Confidentiality

Genetic information about one individual may have implications for other family members and agreement should always be sought before disclosure of such information. If a patient refuses to allow this, his or her wish would normally be respected. Exceptionally, the genetic counsellor may decide to breach confidentiality, when the potential harm to another family member outweighs that to those first considered. Breach of confidence is, however, never undertaken lightly and not without considerable negotiation. The World Health Organization considers the counsellee to have a moral obligation to inform relatives if this allows them in turn to choose whether or not to be screened.

*Genetic information should never be disclosed to third parties, such as insurance companies and employers, without the subject's written consent.*

# 35 Pedigree drawing

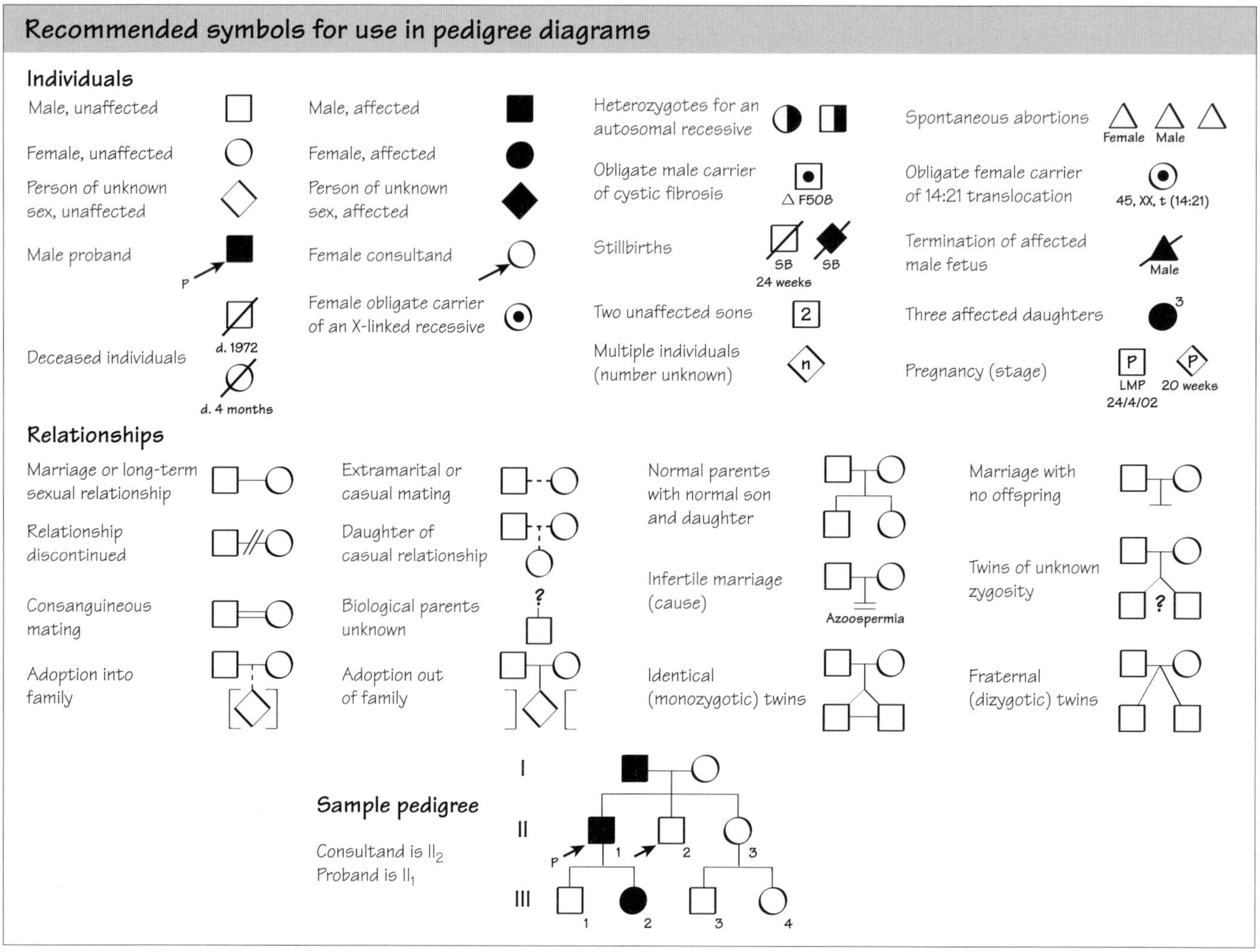

## Recommended symbols for use in pedigree diagrams

### Individuals

Male, unaffected □
Male, affected ■
Heterozygotes for an autosomal recessive ◐ ▮
Spontaneous abortions △ △ △ (Female Male)

Female, unaffected ○
Female, affected ●
Obligate male carrier of cystic fibrosis △ F508
Obligate female carrier of 14:21 translocation ⊙ 45, XX, t (14:21)

Person of unknown sex, unaffected ◇
Person of unknown sex, affected ◆
Stillbirths (SB 24 weeks) (SB)
Termination of affected male fetus ▲ Male

Male proband ■ P
Female consultand ○
Two unaffected sons [2]
Three affected daughters ●³

Deceased individuals ⧄ d. 1972 / ⦸ d. 4 months
Female obligate carrier of an X-linked recessive ⊙
Multiple individuals (number unknown) ◇n
Pregnancy (stage) [P] LMP 24/4/02    ◇P 20 weeks

### Relationships

Marriage or long-term sexual relationship □—○
Extramarital or casual mating □--○
Normal parents with normal son and daughter
Marriage with no offspring □⊤○

Relationship discontinued □//○
Daughter of casual relationship □ ⋮ ○
Infertile marriage (cause) Azoospermia
Twins of unknown zygosity □ ? ○

Consanguineous mating □═○
Biological parents unknown ?
Identical (monozygotic) twins
Fraternal (dizygotic) twins

Adoption into family □⋮○
Adoption out of family

### Sample pedigree

Consultand is II₂
Proband is II₁

I
II    P → ■ 1   → 2   3
III   1  ●2  3  4

## Overview

The collection of information about a family is the first and most important step taken by doctors and nurses when providing genetic counselling. A clear and unambiguous **pedigree diagram**, or 'family tree', provides a permanent record of the most pertinent information and is the best aid to clear thinking about family relationships.

Information is usually collected initially from the **consultand**, i.e. the person requesting genetic advice. If other family members need to be approached it may be wise to advise them in advance of the information required.

The affected individual who caused the consultand(s) to seek advice is called the **propositus** (male), **proposita** (female), **proband** or **index case**. The latter is frequently a child or more distant relative, or the consultand may also be the proband. A standard medical history is required for the proband and all other affected family members.

## Rules for pedigree diagrams

A sample pedigree is shown in the figure (see also Chapters 17–20). Females are symbolized by circles, males by squares and persons of unknown sex by diamonds. Affected individuals are represented by solid symbols, those unaffected by open symbols. Marriages or matings are indicated by horizontal lines linking male and female symbols, with the male partner preferably to the left. Offspring are shown beneath the parental symbols, in birth order from left to right, linked to the mating line by a vertical, and numbered (1, 2, 3, etc.), from left to right in

Arabic numerals. The generations are indicated in Roman numerals (I, II, III, etc.), from top to bottom on the left, with the earliest generation labelled I.

The proband is indicated by an arrow with the letter P, the consultand by an arrow alone. (N.B. earlier practice was to indicate the proband by an arrow without the P).

Only conventional symbols should be used, but it is admissible (and recommended) to annotate diagrams with more complex information. If there are details that could cause embarrassment (e.g. illegitimacy or extra-marital paternity) these should be recorded as supplementary notes.

Include the contact address and telephone number of the consultand on supplementary notes. Add the same details for each additional individual that needs to be contacted.

The compiler of the family tree should record the date it was compiled and append their name or initials.

**Table 35.1** Autosomal dominant diseases.

| Autosomal dominant diseases | Frequency/ 1000 births* |
|---|---|
| 1 Dominant otosclerosis (progressive deafness due to bony overgrowth in inner ear) | 3.00 |
| 2 Familial hypercholesterolaemia (raised levels of blood cholesterol) | 2.00 |
| 3 Dentinogenesis imperfecta (failure of formation of tooth dentine) | 1.20 |
| 4 Adult polycystic kidney disease | 1.00 |
| 5 Multiple exostoses (bony growths on bone surfaces) | 0.50 |
| 6 Huntington disease (progressive degeneration of central nervous system) | 0.50 |
| 7 Neurofibromatosis (tumour-like growths in skin and nervous system) | 0.40 |
| 8 Myotonic dystrophy (severe atrophy of certain muscles) | 0.20 |
| 9 Congenital spherocytosis (haemolytic anaemia with spheroidal red blood cells) | 0.20 |
| 10 Achondroplasia (see Chapter 17) | 0.20 |
| 11 Marfan syndrome (see Chapter 17) | 0.10 |
| 12 Familial adenomatous polyposis coli (precancerous growths in large intestine) | 0.10 |
| 13 Dominant blindness | 0.10 |
| 14 Dominant congenital deafness | 0.10 |
| 15 Others | ~2.00 |
| **Total** | ~11.5/1000 |

*Frequency in Europeans.

**Table 35.2** Autosomal recessive diseases.

| Autosomal recessive diseases | Frequency/ 10000 births* |
|---|---|
| 1 Cystic fibrosis (see Chapter 18) | 0.50 |
| 2 Recessive mental retardation | 0.50 |
| 3 Congenital deafness | 0.20 |
| 4 Phenylketonuria (see Chapter 18) | 0.10 |
| 5 Spinal muscular atrophy (see Chapter 18) | 0.10 |
| 6 Recessive blindness | 0.10 |
| 7 Congenital adrenal hyperplasia (causes virilization of females) | 0.10 |
| 8 Others | ~0.30 |
| **Total** | ~2/1000 |

## The practical approach

1 Start your drawing in the middle of the page.
2 Aim to collect details on three (or more) generations.
3 Ask specifically about:
  (a) consanguinity of partners;
  (b) miscarriages;
  (c) terminated pregnancies;
  (d) stillbirths;
  (e) neonatal and infant deaths;
  (f) handicapped or malformed children;
  (g) multiple partnerships;
  (h) deceased relatives.
4 Be aware of potentially sensitive issues such as adoption and wrongly ascribed paternity.
5 To simplify the diagram unrelated marriage partners may be omitted, but a note should be made whether their phenotype is normal or unknown.
6 Sibs of similar phenotype may be represented as one symbol, with a number to indicate how many are in that category.

The details below should be inserted beside each symbol, whether that individual is alive or dead. Personal details of normal individuals should also be specified. The ethnic background of the family should be recorded if it is different from that of the main population.
1 Full name (including maiden name).
2 Date of birth.
3 Date and cause of death.
4 Any specific medical diagnosis.

## Uses of pedigrees

A good pedigree can reveal the mode of inheritance of a monogenic disease (see Tables 35.1–35.4 and Chapters 17–20) and can be used to predict the genetic risk in several instances. These include:
1 the current pregnancy;
2 the risk for future offspring of those parents (**recurrence risk**);
3 the risk of disease among offspring of close relatives.
4 the probability of adult disease, in cases of diseases of late onset.

**Table 35.3** X-linked recessive diseases.

| X-linked recessive diseases | Frequency/10000 male births |
|---|---|
| G6PD deficiency (geographically very variable) | 0–6500 |
| Red and green colour blindness | 800 |
| Fragile X syndrome | 5.0 |
| Non-specific X-linked mental retardation | 5.0 |
| Duchenne muscular dystrophy | 3.0 |
| Haemophilia A | 2.0 |
| Becker muscular dystrophy | 0.5 |
| Haemophilia B | 0.3 |
| Agammaglobulinaemia (X-linked) | 0.1 |

**Table 35.4** X-linked dominant diseases.

| |
|---|
| Hypophosphataemia (vitamin D resistant rickets) |
| Incontinentia pigmenti (lethal in males) |
| Rett syndrome (lethal in males) |
| Oro–facio–digital syndrome |

## Risk assessment in X-linked recessive disease: Duchenne muscular dystrophy

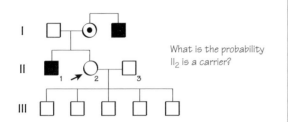

What is the probability II₂ is a carrier?

| Probabilities | II₂ has inherited disease allele | II₂ has not inherited disease allele |
|---|---|---|
| Prior | $\dfrac{1}{2}$ | $\dfrac{1}{2}$ |
| Conditional | $\left(\dfrac{1}{2}\right)^5 = \dfrac{1}{32}$ | $1$ |
| Joint | $\dfrac{1}{2} \times \dfrac{1}{32} = \dfrac{1}{64}$ | $1 \times \dfrac{1}{2} = \dfrac{1}{2} = \dfrac{32}{64}$ |
| Posterior | $\dfrac{\frac{1}{64}}{\frac{1}{64} + \frac{32}{64}} = \dfrac{1}{64} \times \dfrac{64}{33} = \dfrac{1}{33}$ | |

## Risk assessment in autosomal recessive disease: cystic fibrosis

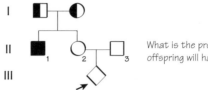

What is the probability the indicated offspring will have CF?

| Probabilities | II-3 is a CF carrier | | II-3 is not a CF carrier |
|---|---|---|---|
| Prior | $\dfrac{1}{20}$ | (carrier frequency) | $\dfrac{19}{20}$ |
| Conditional | $\dfrac{1}{10}$ | (deficiency in screening tests) | $1$ |
| Joint | $\dfrac{1}{20} \times \dfrac{1}{10} = \dfrac{1}{200}$ | | $1 \times \dfrac{19}{20} = \dfrac{19}{20} = \dfrac{190}{200}$ |
| Posterior | $\dfrac{\frac{1}{200}}{\frac{1}{200} + \frac{190}{200}} = \dfrac{1}{200} \times \dfrac{200}{191} = \dfrac{1}{191}$ | | |

Final posterior probability child will be a CF homozygote:

$$= \dfrac{2}{3} \times \dfrac{1}{191} \times \dfrac{1}{4} = \dfrac{1}{1146}$$

## Risk assessment in autosomal dominant disease of incomplete penetrance: familial retinoblastoma ($P = 0.8$; see Chapter 32)

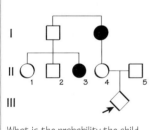

What is the probability the child of II-4 will have retinoblastoma?

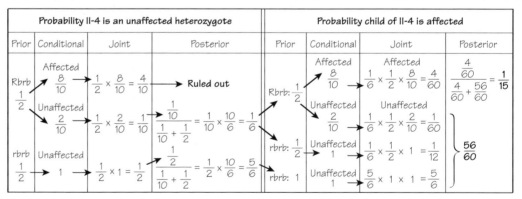

| | Probability II-4 is an unaffected heterozygote | | | | Probability child of II-4 is affected | | | |
|---|---|---|---|---|---|---|---|---|
| | Prior | Conditional | Joint | Posterior | Prior | Conditional | Joint | Posterior |
| Rbrb | $\dfrac{1}{2}$ | Affected $\dfrac{8}{10}$ | $\dfrac{1}{2} \times \dfrac{8}{10} = \dfrac{4}{10}$ | Ruled out | Rbrb: $\dfrac{1}{2}$ | Affected $\dfrac{8}{10}$ | Affected $\dfrac{1}{6} \times \dfrac{1}{2} \times \dfrac{8}{10} = \dfrac{4}{60}$ | $\dfrac{\frac{4}{60}}{\frac{4}{60} + \frac{56}{60}} = \dfrac{1}{15}$ |
| | | Unaffected $\dfrac{2}{10}$ | $\dfrac{1}{2} \times \dfrac{2}{10} = \dfrac{1}{10}$ | $\dfrac{\frac{1}{10}}{\frac{1}{10} + \frac{1}{2}} = \dfrac{1}{10} \times \dfrac{10}{6} = \dfrac{1}{6}$ | | Unaffected $\dfrac{2}{10}$ | Unaffected $\dfrac{1}{6} \times \dfrac{1}{2} \times \dfrac{2}{10} = \dfrac{1}{60}$ | |
| rbrb | $\dfrac{1}{2}$ | Unaffected $1$ | $\dfrac{1}{2} \times 1 = \dfrac{1}{2}$ | $\dfrac{\frac{1}{2}}{\frac{1}{10} + \frac{1}{2}} = \dfrac{1}{2} \times \dfrac{10}{6} = \dfrac{5}{6}$ | rbrb: $\dfrac{1}{2}$ | Unaffected $1$ | $\dfrac{1}{6} \times \dfrac{1}{2} \times 1 = \dfrac{1}{12}$ | $\dfrac{56}{60}$ |
| | | | | | rbrb: $1$ | Unaffected $1$ | $\dfrac{5}{6} \times 1 \times 1 = \dfrac{5}{6}$ | |

## Overview

A major part of the burden of a genetic disorder is the risk of recurrence in the family. A prime goal of assessment therefore is to estimate the risk of transmission by the same couple to later children and by affected and unaffected family members to their children. The simple application of Mendelian theory can often provide a rough guide, but such estimates generally need to be refined by inclusion of other considerations such as penetrance. This is most readily achieved by application of Bayes' theorem.

## Risk assessment

A combination of several factors is used to determine the basic risk of transmission of a genetic disorder (see Chapter 40):

**1 Diagnosis.** A correct diagnosis is critical for the accurate assessment of genetic risks. Correct diagnosis may indicate not only the mode of inheritance, but also suggest appropriate carrier and/or prenatal diagnostic tests.

**2 Family history.** Even in the absence of a diagnosis, assessment of the family history may reveal the pattern of transmission and provide clues to penetrance (Chapter 35).

**3 Ethnic background**. Certain ethnic groups are known to be at increased risk for specific genetic traits (see Chapters 23, 25 and 34), so providing guidance for assessment of carrier status and prenatal diagnosis.

## Application of Bayes' theorem

### X-linked recessive disease

Consider a woman with both a brother and an uncle with X-linked Duchenne muscular dystrophy (see figure ); since her mother must be a carrier (i.e. is an '**obligate carrier**'), the woman has a 50% chance of also being a carrier. This corresponds to her '**prior probability**' of being a carrier. However, if, for example, she has had five unaffected sons we can use this fact to recalculate the '**conditional probability**' of her carrier status and then the **relative likelihood** that she is, rather than is not, a carrier.

Prior probabilities are generally calculated from the pedigree. The prior probability of this woman being a carrier is 1/2 and that she would have five unaffected sons, given that she *is* a carrier, is $(1/2)^5 = 1/32$. The prior probability of her *not* being a carrier is also 1/2, and, if so, the conditional probability of having five normal sons is 1. The product of the prior and conditional probabilities is the '**joint probability**'; in this case 1/64 and 1/2, respectively.

The **relative likelihood** of her being a carrier, also known as the '**posterior probability**', is calculated as the joint probability of her being a carrier divided by the sum of the two joint probabilities.

In mathematical terms this is:

$$\frac{1/64}{(1/64 + 1/2)} = 1/33$$

This calculation is an example of the application of **Bayes' theorem**, commonly used in this context as it allows incorporation of such factors as age-related onset of disease, incomplete penetrance and the results of genetic testing.

### Autosomal recessive disease

The risk of recessive disease depends on coincidence of three circumstances: mother being a carrier, father being a carrier and child inheriting both disease alleles.

Consider a phenotypically normal woman whose brother has cystic fibrosis (CF) (see figure). She is married to a Northern European man and wishes to know the chance their planned child will have CF. The carrier risk for CF among Northern Europeans is around 1/20 and there are laboratory DNA tests for 90% of all CF mutations. The tests on him yield negative results, making his posterior probability of being a carrier 1/191 (see figure).

In matings between two heterozygotes we expect normal homozygotes, heterozygotes and mutant homozygotes in the ratio $1:2:1$. Since this woman is unaffected, she is either a normal homozygote (CF/CF; initial probability 0.25) or a heterozygote (CF/cf; initial probability 0.5). Her probability of being a carrier is therefore $0.5/(0.5 + 0.25) = 2/3$. The final posterior probability of their having a child with CF is therefore $2/3 \times 1/191 \times 1/4 = 1/1146$.

This example is given to illustrate application of the theory, in a real situation of course the woman would usually also be tested, so reducing the range of possibilities and refining the estimate of risk.

### Autosomal dominant of incomplete penetrance

Familial retinoblastoma is transmitted as a dominant of penetrance ($P$) $= 0.8$ (see Chapter 32). As shown diagrammatically in the figure, the posterior probability of the child of an unaffected suspected carrier (Rb/rb) being affected is 1/15.

## Application of empiric risks

Risks are currently not calculable for some conditions, such as multifactorial disease; instead we refer to tables of **empiric risks**, i.e. observed incidences (Table 40.1).

## Isolated cases

Congenital deafness frequently occurs in families in which there have been no previous cases. In such instances risk is based on the observation that 70% of cases of deafness are genetic, of which 2/3 are recessive. On the assumption it probably is inherited and recessive, risk of recurrence is calculated as $7/10 \times 2/3 \times 1/4 = 1/9$.

## Difficulties

Patterns of inheritance may be obscured by small size of the sibship, by new mutation, or by failure of some genotypes to survive to birth. There can also be diagnostic difficulties due to absent or variable gene expression, or lack of accurate information on absent family members.

Even if a genetic disorder occurs in one family member only, it may be possible to deduce the probable mode of inheritance by comparison with other families that show identical symptoms. However, it should be remembered that many conditions are **genetically heterogeneous**, i.e. disorders that are clinically indistinguishable may be caused by more than one genetic lesion, which may follow different patterns of inheritance. In such cases ethnic background can be informative. Conversely, members of the same family may display variant manifestations of the same condition, as with Marfan syndrome (see Chapter 17).

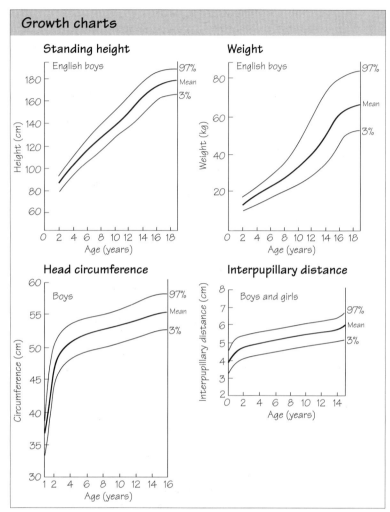

**Growth charts**

Standing height — English boys — 97% Mean 3% — Height (cm) / Age (years)

Weight — English boys — 97% Mean 3% — Weight (kg) / Age (years)

Head circumference — Boys — 97% Mean 3% — Circumference (cm) / Age (years)

Interpupillary distance — Boys and girls — 97% Mean 3% — Interpupillary distance (cm) / Age (years)

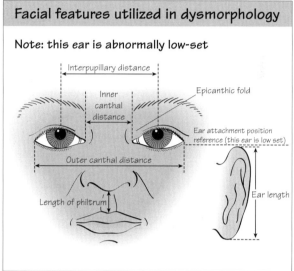

**Facial features utilized in dysmorphology**

Note: this ear is abnormally low-set

Interpupillary distance — Inner canthal distance — Epicanthic fold — Ear attachment position reference (this ear is low set) — Outer canthal distance — Length of philtrum — Ear length

**Table 37.1**
**Some well-recognized malformation syndromes**

| | |
|---|---|
| Apert syndrome (acrocephalosyndactyly) | Edward syndrome |
| Beckwith–Wiedemann syndrome | Fragile X syndrome |
| | Noonan syndrome |
| CHARGE association | Patau syndrome |
| Cleidocranial dysostosis | Rubinstein–Taybi syndrome |
| Cri-du-chat syndrome | Smith–Lemli–Opitz syndrome |
| Crouzon disease (craniofacial dysostosis) | Treacher Collins syndrome (mandibulofacial dysostosis) |
| De Lange syndrome | Turner syndrome |
| Di George syndrome | VATER association |
| Down syndrome | Williams syndrome |
| | Wolf–Hirschhorn syndrome |

## Overview

Anatomical features are considered **dysmorphic** if their measures lie outside the normal range. **Dysmorphology** is the discipline concerned with their identification, delineation, diagnosis and management.

Quantitative characters vary with age and sex, but measures of different features in a normal subject should all lie within the same part of their respective ranges. An exceptional measure reflects abnormality. Since some dysmorphic features relate to age, re-examination at a later date can be helpful.

Two to four per cent of newborn babies have a physical anomaly and currently over 2000 diagnoses are listed. Multiple dysmorphic features enable identification of known syndromes. For example **fetal alcohol syndrome**, present in 1/300–1/1000 children, is indicated by the combination of growth deficiency, microcephaly (small head), short palpebral fissures (eye slits), a smooth philtrum (channel in upper lip) and a thin upper lip.

## Classification of abnormal developmental features

A variety of congenital anomalies have been delineated, the understanding of which is important in providing counselling to families (see Chapter 21). These are classified as follows:

1 **Malformations**, e.g. polydactyly (presence of extra fingers or toes).
2 **Deformations**, e.g. moulding of the fetal head due to uterine fibroids.
3 **Disruptions**, e.g. amputation of a limb due to entrapment by an amniotic band.
4 **Dysplasias**, e.g. neuronal **heterotopia** (i.e. presence of normal tissue at abnormal sites) in the brain.

Malformations may also be classified in terms of occurrence of features.

1 **Isolated malformation**, e.g. extra digit on one hand.
2 **Sequence**, e.g. cleft palate in infant with under-development of the jaw (**Pierre–Robin sequence**), in which upward displacement of the tongue in a very small mouth interferes with palatal closure.

**3 Association**: tendency of multiple malformations to occur together non-randomly, usually for unknown reasons, e.g. **VATER association**, in which **v**ertebral and **a**nal anomalies, **t**racheo-**e**sophageal fistula, and **r**adial anomalies occur together in various combinations and **VACTERL association**, which also includes **c**ardiac and **l**imb defects.

**4 Syndrome**: a set of phenotypic features that frequently occur together as a characteristic of a disease, e.g. Down syndrome.

## Clinically important growth parameters

Human growth charts show mean values and ranges plotted against age. Individuals who lie outside the 3rd and 97th centiles are considered abnormal. Assessment of infants requires careful physical examination, photographic records and history taking.

The following measures may be taken if there are specific concerns about disproportionate growth.

1 Standing height:
   (a) overall height;
   (b) lower segment: floor to upper border of pubis;
   (c) upper segment: overall height minus lower segment.
2 Sitting height.
3 Linear growth, i.e. change in body length over time.
4 Arm span.
5 Weight.
6 Head circumference: maximum occipitofrontal circumference is an indirect measure of brain size:
   (a) **microcephaly** can reflect poor brain growth or premature fusion of skull sutures;
   (b) **macrocephaly** may indicate high intracranial fluid pressure.
7 Eyes:
   (a) **hypertelorism** is a feature of nearly 400 syndromes, describing abnormally widely spaced orbits;
   (b) **hypotelorism** refers to abnormally closely spaced orbits, found in some 40 syndromes;
   (c) **telecanthus** refers to an increase in the distance between the inner canthi with normal interorbital distance and is a feature of around 90 syndromes;
   (d) **blepharophimosis** is reduction in the length of the palpebral fissures and features in over 100 syndromes;
   (e) **epicanthic folds** are skin folds over the inner canthi;
   (f) **upwards slant** of the eyes means that the inner canthi are lower than the outer, as in Down syndrome (see Chapter 14);
   (g) **downwards slant** describes eyes with the inner canthi higher than the outer, as in Cri-du-chat syndrome (see Chapter 15).
8 Ears: maximum ear length and ear position are recorded. Ears are described as low-set if the upper border of their attachment is below a line through the outer canthi and the occipital protuberance at the back of the skull.
9 Head shape:
   (a) **brachycephaly** describes short anteroposterior skull length;
   (b) **dolichocephaly** refers to long anteroposterior skull length.
10 Testicular volume.
11 Limbs:
   (a) **syndactyly** indicates digital fusion, osseous (**synphalangism**), or cutaneous (**webbing**);
   (b) **polydactyly** describes extra digits on the **preaxial** (radial/tibial), or **postaxial** (ulnar/fibular) side;
   (c) **clinodactyly** describes an incurved digit, most often the fifth finger (see Down syndrome, Chapter 14).

## Diagnosis in dysmorphology

Correct classification of congenital anomalies has implications for diagnosis and hence for management, prognosis and counselling. Tissue samples should be taken from malformed stillbirths and fetuses for laboratory investigation.

A systematic approach to diagnosis would involve the following:

**1 Family pedigree construction** (see Chapter 35).
**2 Pregnancy history**. Record drug exposure (e.g. treatment for maternal epilepsy), excess alcohol intake, maternal physiological disorders such as diabetes and infection (see Chapter 11).
**3 Physical examination**.
**4 Laboratory investigations**, e.g. chromosome analysis, skeletal survey or brain imaging.
**5 Differential diagnosis**. Illustrated texts and computerized databases can be used for reference (see Appendix).
**6 Conclusion**. Currently in perhaps 50% of cases a secure diagnosis cannot be reached.

## G-banding and labelling of chromosomes

Chromosome 7 is shown at resolutions of 450, 550 and 850 bands per haploid set. The indicated band is designated 7q31.32

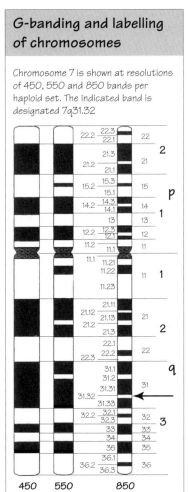

450    550    850

## Three chromosome forms (alternative representation, at metaphase)

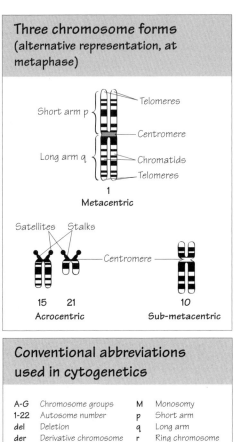

## Conventional abbreviations used in cytogenetics

| A-G | Chromosome groups | M | Monosomy |
|-----|-------------------|---|----------|
| 1-22 | Autosome number | p | Short arm |
| del | Deletion | q | Long arm |
| der | Derivative chromosome | r | Ring chromosome |
| dup | Duplication | t | Translocation |
| i | Isochromosome | T | Trisomy |
| ins | Insertion | ter | Terminal |
| inv | Inversion | | |

## Use of FISH probes

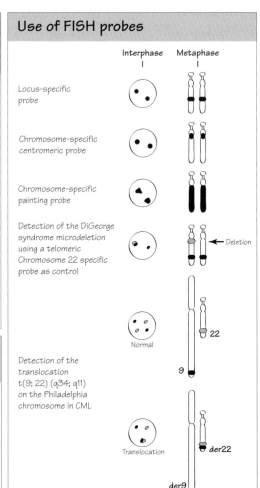

## Overview

The microscopic study of chromosomes is called **cytogenetics**. Traditionally it is performed on compacted chromosomes at a magnification of about 1000, providing resolution to around 3 million base pairs, or one narrow chromosome band (see Chapter 3). By incorporation of molecular techniques this can be reduced to 10 kb.

Conventional cytogenetics uses mitotic chromosomes. The chorion (**syncytiotrophoblast**) and bone-marrow normally contain sufficient dividing cells for examination, but most tissues require culturing *in vitro*, with an overall time schedule of about 10 days. **Molecular cytogenetics** utilizing DNA probes can be applied directly to interphase nuclei.

## Preparation of a karyotype

A visual karyotype is prepared by arresting dividing cells at metaphase with a spindle inhibitor such as *colchicine* (see Chapter 9), spreading the cells on a glass slide and staining with Giemsa stain. Traditionally a photographic positive is then made and the chromosomes cut out and assembled on a card in pairs in order of size, sometimes in conventional groups

A-E (see Chapter 42). In modern practice, the latter step is replaced by digital imaging. Chromosomes 1, 3, 16, 19 and 20, with the centromere in the middle, are known as **metacentric**; 13, 14, 15, 21, 22, and Y, with the centromere near one end, are **acrocentric**. The rest are **submetacentric**. The short arm is symbolized 'p' (for petite) and the long arm 'q'.

**Karyotype formulae** are described in Chapter 14. Positions of genes along chromosome arms are defined by **region** number (from the centromere outwards), **band**, **sub-band** and **sub-sub-band** numbers, e.g. 12q24.32 refers to Chromosome 12, long arm, region 2, band 4, sub-band 3, sub-sub-band 2. **High-resolution banding** involves fixation before the chromosomes are fully compacted.

**C-banding** stains heterochromatin, **NOR staining** reveals the *n*ucleolar *o*rganizer *r*egions on the satellite stalks of the acrocentrics.

## Fluorescence *in situ* hybridization (FISH)

**FISH** enables the specific localization of genes and the direct visualization of abnormalities at the molecular level. With chromosome-specific probes it allows rapid diagnosis or exclusion of trisomy in amniotic fluid cells.

In a typical application, a labelled probe is denatured by heating, added to a metaphase chromosome spread on a microscope slide and incubated overnight to permit sequence-specific hybridization. Surplus probe is then washed off and the bound probe located by overlaying the spread with a solution of fluorescent 'reporter molecule'. Unbound reporter is washed off and a counterstain applied to reveal the chromosomes. Bound reporter, and hence the site of the gene of interest, is then located by its fluorescence under UV light.

The key to this method is the creation of a probe and fluorescent reporter molecule with mutual affinity. This is usually done by exploiting the natural affinity of avidin (a component of hen egg albumin) for the B vitamin, biotin. Probe preparation involves incorporation of biotin-16-dUTP into its DNA, as an analogue of thymidine, during an enzyme-based process akin to DNA repair, called nick translation. The fluorescent marker is derived by direct conjugation of avidin with a fluorescent dye.

Amplification of the fluorescent signal can be achieved by overlaying with further layers of biotin and fluorescent avidin.

## Use of unique sequence probes
### Microdeletions
Submicroscopic deletions can be detected with fluorescent probes directed against one or more unique sequences within the deleted interval (see Table 38.1).

Table 38.1 Examples of syndromes associated with microdeletions, in approximate order of decreasing frequency.

| Syndrome | Site of deletion |
|---|---|
| DiGeorge/velocardiofacial | 22q11 |
| Williams | 7q11.23 |
| Smith–Magenis | 17p11.2 |
| Prader–Willi | 15q11 (paternal) |
| Angelman | 15q11 (maternal) |
| Wolf–Hirschhorn | 4p16.3 |
| Langer–Giedion | 8q24.1 |
| Rubinstein–Taybi | 16p |
| Alpha-thalassaemia and mental retardation | 16p13.3 |
| Miller–Dieker lissencephaly | 17p13.3 |
| Alagille | 20p11 |
| WAGR (Wilm's tumour, aniridia, genital, retardation) | 11p13 |
| Retinoblastoma | 13q14.1 |

### Translocations
FISH probes directed at the *BCR* and *abl* sequences can be used to reveal the Philadelphia chromosome (see Chapter 31) as two adjacent fluorescent signals on the derivative Chromosome 22. FISH probes to regions near the telomeres can be useful in identifying subtelomeric rearrangements resulting in unbalanced karyotypes that may lead to mental retardation.

### Sex chromosome rearrangements
In some phenotypic males lacking a Y chromosome, an SRY probe reveals the site to which the male. Determining *SRY* locus (see Chapter 12) has been translocated from its normal site at Yp11, often to the X.

## Subtelomeric, centromeric and repeat sequence probes
Probes directed at chromosome-specific subtelomeric sequences, centromeric alphoid and beta-satellite repeats and other moderately repetitive sequences are useful for chromosome identification and detecting aneuploidy and structural rearrangements.

## Chromosome painting
When unique sequence probes for a single chromosome are pooled and labelled with the same fluorochrome this creates a 'chromosome paint' that identifies that specific chromosome or its fragments after translocation (see book cover).

In reverse painting, a battery of probes is made from an *abnormal* chromosome and hybridized to normal metaphase spreads, so allowing the derivation of the abnormal chromosome to be deduced. Such probes are created by assembling many copies of the abnormal chromosome using a fluorescence activated chromosome sorter (see Chapter 28) or microdissection.

## Primed *in situ* hybridization
Primed *in situ* hybridization (PRINZ) technique involves setting up a PCR reaction *in situ* on a chromosome spread. Primers are added that define a specific genetic locus, resulting in a build up of target DNA at the site of interest. If a fluorescent base analogue is incorporated during the PCR reaction the sequence is rendered visible in one step.

## Mendelian disorders with cytogenetic effects
Several single-gene disorders are indicated by abnormalities detectable cytogenetically in special preparations (Table 38.2).

Table 38.2 Single gene disorders with cytogenetic effects.

| Disorder | Inheritance | Cytogenetic effect |
|---|---|---|
| Ataxia telangiectasia | AR | Chromatid damage due to defective DNA repair |
| Bloom syndrome | AR | High frequency of sister chromatid exchange |
| Fanconi anaemia | AR | Chromosome breakage and translocation |
| Fragile X syndrome | X-linked | Chromosome breakage at Xq27.3 |
| Roberts syndrome | AR | Separation of centromeres at metaphase |
| Xeroderma pigmentosum | AR | Defective repair of UV damage, sister chromatid exchange |

## Cancer cytogenetics
Over 150 non-random chromosome changes are associated with neoplasia.

## Indications for chromosome analysis
The following are situations in which cytogenetic investigation is advised.
1 Suspected chromosome abnormality.
2 Multiple congenital anomalies and/or developmental retardation.
3 Disorders of sexual function.
4 Undiagnosed mental retardation.
5 Certain malignancies.
6 Infertility or multiple miscarriage.
7 Stillbirth or neonatal death.

## The basis for biochemical, chemical, bacteriological and DNA screening for phenylketonuria
Sites of action of the alleles for oculocutaneous albinism and congenital hypothyroidism are also shown

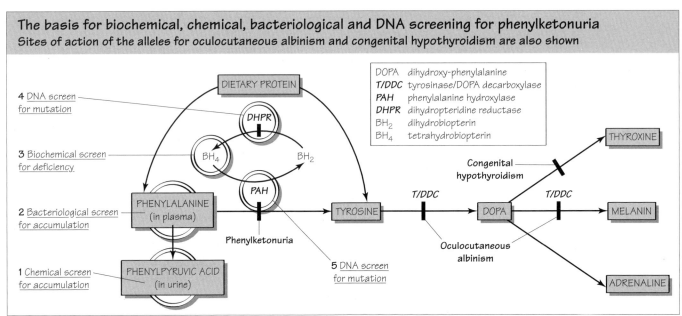

## Enzymatic defects in lysosomal storage disorders
The activities of the indicated enzymes are measured in screening for disease

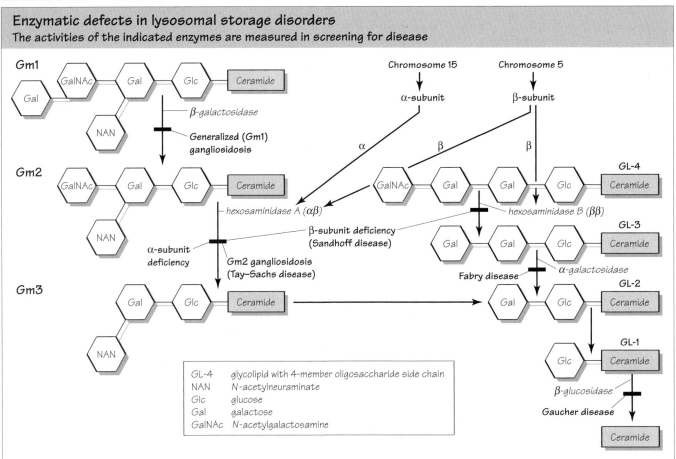

## Overview

'Inborn errors of metabolism' result from mutations in genes that encode enzymes responsible for catalysing biochemical reactions. Clinical disorders arise from abnormal **accumulation of substrate** and/or **deficiency of product**. Diagnosis can be accomplished by detection of accumulated metabolites, enzyme assay, or direct detection of gene mutations. In many instances treatment is available based on **dietary modification**, **coenzyme supplementation**, or **enzyme replacement** (see Chapter 48). **Newborn screening**, aimed at early diagnosis, is carried out in most developed countries, so that treatment can be instituted before the onset of irreversible damage.

## Inborn errors of metabolism

Most inborn errors are recessively inherited, since a 50% level of enzyme activity in heterozygotes is usually sufficient to support normal activity of the biochemical pathway.

The prototypical inborn error is **phenylketonuria** (**PKU**; see Chapter 18) due to a block in the conversion of phenylalanine to tyrosine. In most individuals this involves mutation in the gene that encodes **phenylalanine hydroxylase**. Rarely (1–3%), it may be due to deficiency in one of the enzymes (e.g. dihydropteridine reductase, DHPR) required to synthesize **tetrahydrobiopterin**, which serves as a cofactor in the reaction. Either way, phenylalanine and its derivatives (mainly phenylpyruvic acid) build up to toxic levels, with ensuing irreversible damage to the central nervous system. There is also a deficiency of tyrosine, leading to reduced production of downstream products including melanin, resulting in hypopigmentation, and dihydroxy-phenylalanine (DOPA) possibly contributing to hormonal and neurological dysfunction. The disorder requires screening postnatally, since phenylalanine does not begin to accumulate until after birth (phenylalanine is cleared through the placenta *in utero*). Fortunately, dietary restriction of phenylalanine and supplementation with tyrosine avoids most of the complications of the disorder.

As exemplified by PKU, metabolic disorders can result from mutations in genes that encode enzymes, or in pathways that lead to production of essential cofactors. Accumulated substrate may be toxic, as for phenylalanine, methylmalonic acid (which causes severe metabolic acidosis) and ammonia, when there is a block in one of the enzymes of the urea cycle. Enzyme deficiency can result from gene mutations that lead to deficient production, reduced activity, or abnormal trafficking of the enzyme in the cell. In instances of cofactor deficiency, treatment can sometimes be effected by cofactor supplementation, such as with **cobalamin** (**vitamin B12**) in some cases of **methylmalonic acidaemia**.

The **lysosomal storage disorders** result from deficiency of lysosomal acid hydrolases that digest various substrates, including glycosylated membrane phospholipids (see figure). A prototypical example is **Tay–Sachs disease**, in which GM2 ganglioside accumulates in the lysosomes of neurones, due to deficiency of **hexosominidase A**, leading to progressive degeneration of neurological function. Lysosomal storage diseases tend to be progressive, as more and more cells are rendered dysfunctional by accumulated lysosomal material.

Product deficiency is typified by **oculocutaneous albinism**, in which deficiency of **tyrosinase** (**DOPA decarboxylase**) leads to inability to form melanin pigment (see Chapter 18).

## Approaches to diagnosis

### Detection of metabolites

Detection of metabolites is the time-honoured approach to diagnosis, again typified by phenylketonuria, with measurement of phenylalanine in the blood plasma. This approach offers an inexpensive, sensitive, and specific means of diagnosis and is the basis for most newborn screening methods, where low cost and sensitivity are critical.

A limitation of metabolite detection, however, is that for some disorders, metabolites accumulate only episodically. An example is the **organic acid accumulation disorders**, due to blocks in the metabolism of branched chain amino acids. Mild enzyme deficiency can lead to episodes of metabolic crisis in which organic acids build up, but between episodes, blood or urine studies may be unrevealing.

The technology for metabolite detection has undergone significant evolution. In the case of PKU, newborn screening was initially based on the green colour response when ferric chloride ($FeCl_3$) is sprinkled into the baby's wet nappy (diaper). Following this came Guthrie's **bacterial inhibition assay**. Heelprick blood samples impregnated onto discs of filter paper are placed on a lawn of mutant bacteria that cannot grow in the absence of supplemental phenylalanine. A halo of bacterial growth surrounding a disc indicates a high concentration of phenylalanine in that sample.

Quantitative analysis of amino acids can be carried out by **column chromatography**, while organic acids are detected using **gas chromatography** followed by **mass spectrometry**. More recently, samples are analysed using **tandem mass spectrometry**, which permits detection of a wide variety of metabolites. This approach is rapidly being incorporated into both laboratory diagnosis and newborn screening programs.

### Enzyme assay

Enzyme activity can be assayed *in vitro* using either synthetic or natural substrates. This approach is commonly used to diagnose lysosomal storage disorders, where metabolites are trapped within lysosomes and therefore inaccessible to direct assay. Enzyme assay is, for example, the major approach used in screening for hexosaminidase A deficiency in white blood cells of heterozygous carriers of Tay–Sachs disease (see Chapter 18).

Enzyme assay offers the advantage over substrate quantification that heterozygotes may also be identified, although in some cases there is overlap between their activities and those in normal homozygotes.

### DNA diagnosis

Direct detection of gene mutations is increasingly being used as an approach to diagnosis of inborn errors of metabolism. This approach has several advantages. These include the ability to perform testing very early in development and on any nucleated cells, obviating the need to sample tissues that express the enzyme concerned, or accumulate relevant metabolites. It is also highly specific, particularly in detection of clinically unaffected carriers.

DNA based diagnosis is finding increasing use in **carrier detection schemes**, such as the identification of carriers of **Canavan** and **Gaucher diseases**, both found at high frequency in the Ashkenazi Jewish population (see Table 34.1).

## Reproductive options and the management of genetic risk

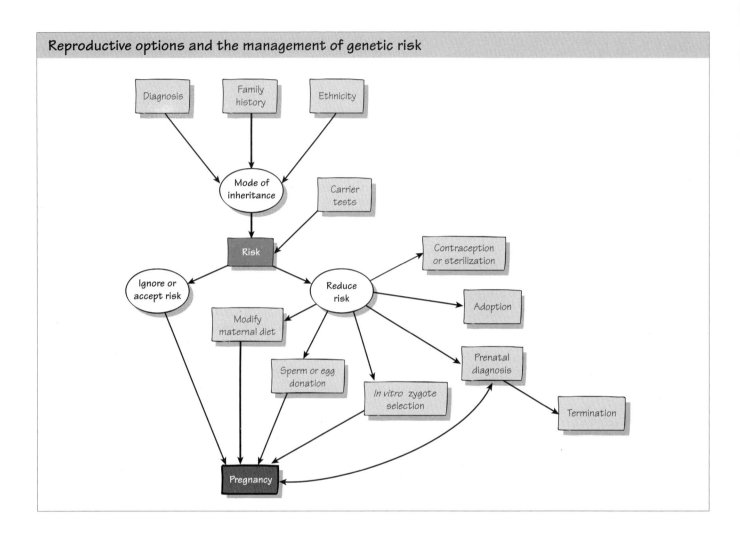

## Overview

Genetic counselling is provided by practitioners with specialist training, both in the principles of genetics and in the processes of communication with patients and families. In essence it involves accurate assessment of the genetic risk associated with reproduction by the couple concerned (see Chapter 36 and Table 40.1), communication of this risk to the consultand(s) and, if necessary, the offer of advice on reproductive options.

*A major tenet of genetic counselling is to be non-directive,* i.e. the personal opinions of the counsellor should not bias the information provided, or create pressure toward a specific management decision. The non-directive approach applies particularly to decisions on prenatal diagnosis, as there is wide divergence of opinion regarding termination of pregnancy. In Britain, legal grounds for termination include 'a substantial risk that if a child were born it would suffer from such physical or mental abnormality as to be seriously handicapped' (UK Abortion Act, 1967). Prenatal diagnostic tests require informed consent, and consultands should be made fully aware of the limitations of such tests.

## The psychological approach

Genetic counselling normally begins with the compilation of a family pedigree. The interview at which this is drawn serves four main purposes:

1 Establishment of rapport between counsellor and consultand.
2 Elucidation of the mode of inheritance of the relevant trait in that family.
3 Collection of information on family relationships, with identification of others at risk.
4 Identification of the consultand's concerns and perceptions of the disease.

As a counsellor you should observe several pointers.
1 Introduce yourself and maintain a warm approach.

**Table 40.1** Empiric recurrence risks % for common multifactorial disorders (From Emery, 1986).

| Disorder | Unaffected parents having a second affected child (%) | Affected parent having an affected child (%) | Affected parent having a second affected child (%) |
|---|---|---|---|
| Asthma | 10 | 26 | — |
| Cleft palate (CP) | 2 | 7 | 15 |
| CL±P | 4 | 4 | 10 |
| Club foot | 3 | 3 | 10 |
| Congenital heart defects | 1–4 | 1–4 | 10 |
| Dislocation of hip | 6 | 12 | 36 |
| Epilepsy (idiopathic) | 5 | 5 | 10 |
| Manic depression | 10–15 | 10–15 | — |
| Pyloric stenosis | | | |
|   Male index case | 2 | 4 | 13 |
|   Female index case | 10 | 17 | 38 |
| Schizophrenia | 10 | 14 | — |
| Spina bifida | 4–5 | 4 | — |

2 When dealing with children provide a toy to occupy them while you speak with the parents.

3 Never *assume* a relationship such as paternity or maternity.

4 Be aware that members of the family who have died may not be mentioned unless you specifically ask about them and that their memory may cause distress.

5 Take information from both sides of the family. This may not only reveal additional important facts, but avoids the possible feeling that guilt or blame is directed at one person.

6 While recording the family history watch for clues, such as agitation and the tone of interaction between family members.

## The counselling process

The counselling process can be considered under four headings.

1 **Genetic contribution**. An understanding of the genetic component of the disorder requires integration of clinical diagnosis, family history and the results of laboratory testing. The affected individual and/or other family members should be made aware of the significance of the diagnosis and how genetic factors lead to risk of recurrence.

**Table 40.2** Reproductive hazards in the population at large.

| Condition | Risk | % Risk |
|---|---|---|
| Spontaneous miscarriage | 1 in 6 | 17 |
| Perinatal death | 1 in 30–100 | 1–3 |
| Neonatal death | 1 in 150 | 0.7 |
| Major congenital malformation | 1 in 33 | 3 |
| Minor congenital malformation | 1 in 7 | 14 |
| Serious mental or physical disability | 1 in 50 | 2 |

2 **Natural history of the disorder**. The patient and family must be educated in the disorder and the medical problems to be expected. It is often helpful for them to meet with parents and physicians who care for patients with similar problems.

3 **Management**. Management of genetic disorders includes: **anticipatory guidance**, recognizing possible complications and how these can be prevented or ameliorated; **surveillance** for treatable or preventable complications; and **management of risk**. The latter includes genetic testing to elucidate carrier risk, and education on reproductive options.

4 **Support**. The genetic counsellor should offer both emotional and logistical support in helping the family make reproductive decisions and cope with genetic risk and its associated emotional burdens. It is difficult for most people to see these in perspective, but an appreciation of the magnitude of reproductive risks in general may be gained by reference to data on reproductive hazards in the population at large (Table 40.2).

## Reproductive options

An estimate of risk of disease for a child to be born to the couple concerned is derived from an understanding of the ethnic background of the family, the deduced mode of inheritance of the condition and the results of laboratory tests. Depending on the magnitude of the perceived risk and/or the outlook of the family, the couple may decide to ignore or accept that risk, or take steps to reduce it.

The latter course could involve modification of maternal diet or lifestyle, or aiming for prenatal diagnosis at a later stage, with the option of termination. Other options could include artificial insemination by donor, egg donation, *in vitro* fertilization with embryo selection, and contraception or sterilization combined with adoption of a healthy, unrelated child.

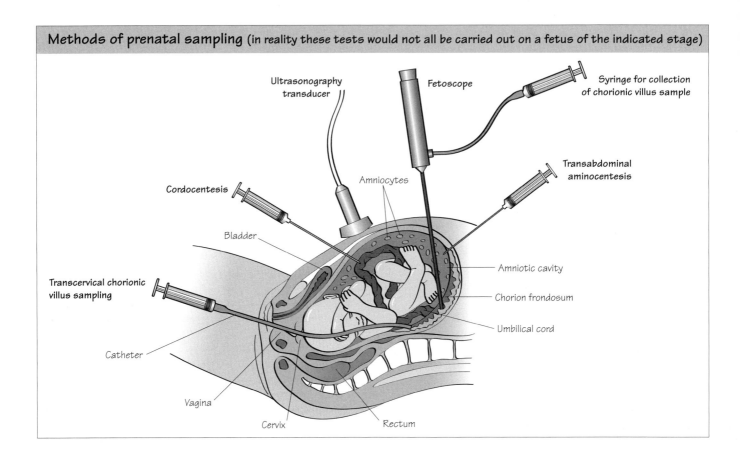

**Methods of prenatal sampling** (in reality these tests would not all be carried out on a fetus of the indicated stage)

## Overview

The term '**prenatal diagnosis**' refers to the diagnosis of genetic disorders in established pregnancies. Such information can guide the family in reproductive decision-making, which may involve terminating the pregnancy, or facilitate planning of appropriate medical, surgical or psychological support. Timing, safety and accuracy are critical.

In North America and Western Europe most pregnant women aged over 35 are offered a dating scan at about 12 weeks and a fetal physical anomaly scan at 18–20 weeks. If there is to be a termination, this is preferable in the first trimester (up to 13 weeks) as this is safer for the mother. There is a generally applied 24-week limit for pregnancy termination in Britain, but the law permits termination for severe abnormalities up to 40 weeks.

## Non-invasive procedures
### Ultrasound scanning

In **ultrasound scanning**, echoes reflected from organ boundaries are converted to images on a monitor. This allows identification of around 300 different malformations, with no known hazard.

Anencephaly can be detected at 10–12 weeks, but for most abnormalities the optimum is 18–20 weeks, when the NTDs, severe skeletal dysplasias, cleft lip and palate, microphthalmia and structural abnormalities of the brain, abdominal organs and heart are usually detectable.

By the third trimester hydrocephalus, microcephaly and duodenal atresia are also detectable.

Obstetric indications for ultrasonography include confirmation of viable or multiple pregnancy, assessment of fetal age and growth, location of the placenta and assessment of amniotic fluid volume. It is an integral aspect of invasive techniques such as **amniocentesis**, **chorionic villus** and **fetal blood sampling**.

### X-rays

Because of the risk of mutagenic injury X-rays should be avoided, although they are sometimes used to assess fetal skeletal dysplasia (see Chapter 29).

### Magnetic resonance imaging

New, fast MRI techniques permit prenatal imaging, useful in the diagnosis of internal anomalies such as brain malformation.

### Screening of maternal blood

Maternal serum can provide useful indicators, e.g. of alpha-fetoprotein (**AFP**), human chorionic gonadotrophin (**hCG**) and **unconjugated oestriol** (**UE3**) in relation to Down syndrome (Chapter 47). Elevated levels of AFP are associated especially with NTDs. Analysis of AFP, hCG and UE3 provide a means of screening for trisomies 18 and 21.

**Table 41.1** Prenatal sampling and associated risks.

| Stage | Optimal time | Risk of miscarriage | Availability |
|---|---|---|---|
| *Preimplantation* | | | |
| Embryo biopsy | 6–10 cell stage | Unknown, presumed safe | Limited |
| *First trimester (0–13 weeks)* | | | |
| Chorionic villus sampling | | | |
|    Transcervical | 9–12 weeks* | 0.5–2.0% | Specialized |
|    Transabdominal | 9–13 weeks* | 0.5–2.0% | Specialized |
| *Second trimester (14–26 weeks)* | | | |
| Placental biopsy | | | |
|    Transabdominal | 14–40 weeks* | 0.5–2.0% | Specialized |
| Ultrasonography | 16–18 weeks | Safe | Widely available |
| Amniocentesis | 16–18 weeks* | 0.5–1.0% | Widely available |
| Cordocentesis | 18–40 weeks* | 1% | Specialized |
| Fetoscopy | 18–20 weeks | 3% | Widely available |
| Fetal tissue biopsy | 18–20 weeks* | 3% | Very specialized |

*When culture of embryonic tissue is necessary diagnosis is delayed by 2–4 weeks.

## Invasive procedures

The accepted guideline for invasive testing is that the risk of a seriously abnormal fetus is at least as great as that of miscarriage from the procedure. **Conditions considered serious include those that lead inevitably to stillbirth or early death, or to children with severe multiple or progressive handicap.** The chief indications for prenatal diagnosis are:

1 Maternal age >35 years at term.
2 Previous child with *de novo* chromosome abnormality.
3 Presence of a recognized chromosome anomaly.
4 Family history of detectable genetic defect.
5 Family history of an X-linked disorder.
6 Elevated serum AFP or family history of NTD.
7 Parental consanguinity in families with recessive disease.
8 Maternal illness, medication, or teratogen exposure.
9 Abnormal amniotic fluid volume.
10 Parents known to be carriers of certain disorders.

Induction of rhesus iso-immunization by invasive procedures in Rh⁻ mothers is prevented by administration of anti-D immunoglobulin.

## Chorionic villus sampling

In chorionic villus sampling (CVS) a **syncytiotrophoblast** biopsy is aspirated via a catheter through the cervix at 10–12 weeks, or by transabdominal puncture at any time up to term, both guided by ultrasonography. The early timing allows diagnosis by about 12 weeks, but there is an associated risk 0.5–2.0% above the spontaneous abortion rate of 7%.

Since syncytiotrophoblast nuclei divide rapidly, karyotyping is possible without culturing, but cultured material provides more reliable results.

## Amniocentesis

Amniocentesis is especially valuable at 16–18 weeks for estimating AFP concentration and acetylcholinesterase activity in pregnancies at risk of NTDs. After prior localization of the placenta by ultrasound, a needle is inserted aseptically through the mother's abdominal wall and into the amniotic cavity, and a 10–20 ml sample is withdrawn. It carries a risk of 0.5–1.0% of causing miscarriage, in addition to the natural risk of 2.5% at 16 weeks, or 7% when AFP levels are high.

Amniotic fluid cells shed from the skin, respiratory and urinary tracts usually require culture prior to karyotyping, fetal sexing or enzyme assay, although 'interphase FISH' (Chapter 38) is now being offered for screening for trisomies and sex chromosome aneuploidies.

## Cordocentesis

From week 18 onwards a fetal blood sample can be taken by inserting a fine needle transabdominally into the umbilical cord. This is carried out with guidance by fetoscopy (with a 3% extra risk of miscarriage) or ultrasonography (with a 1% extra risk). Culture of extracted cells for a few days provides material suitable for chromosome analysis or DNA investigation.

## Fetoscopy

Fetoscopy involves viewing the fetus through an **endoscope** (i.e. an optical fibre). The optimum stage is 18–20 weeks and it carries a risk of fetal loss of 3%. It is used in fetal biopsy, but its most common application is in the investigation of bladder obstruction.

## Embryo biopsy

Fetoscopy enables biopsy collection for prenatal diagnosis of serious skin and liver disorders.

## Preimplantation genetic diagnosis

In the context of *in-vitro* fertilization, one or two cells are collected at the 6–10 cell stage for direct examination by PCR or FISH (see Chapters 38 and 45), enabling selection of healthy embryos for implantation. (Culturing of these cells would contravene the UK Human Fertilization and Embryology Act 1990.)

## Problems of prenatal sampling

True fetal **mosaicism** is found in around 0.25% of fetuses, indicated by discrepant primary cultures. About 1% have **confined placental mosaicism. Maternal cell contamination** is a problem most common in long-term chorionic villus cultures.

# 42 Linkage analysis

## The G-banded human karyotype (Chromosomes are shown at the 550 band level of resolution)

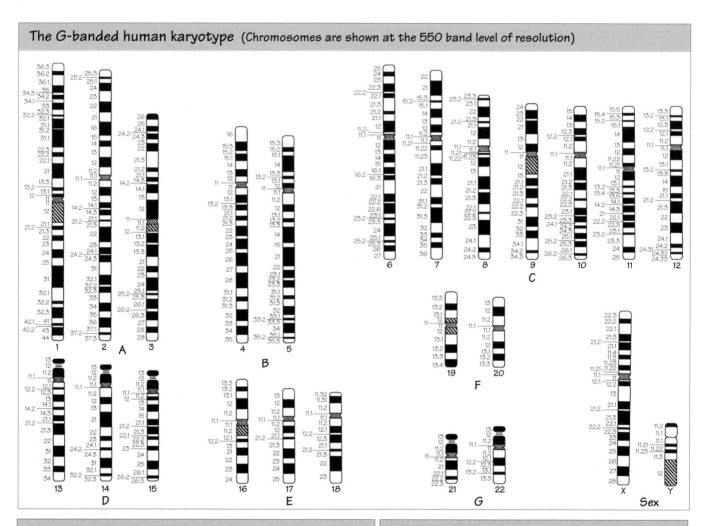

## Linkage analysis in an autosomal dominant disorder

The two alleles at the disease locus are labelled '+' for wildtype and '−' for disease; alleles at marker locus 'A' are labelled '1' and '2'. At the right, the map of the region is shown, as well as the consequence of recombination. Unborn child III-4 has probably (99%) not inherited the '−' allele, but there remains a 1% chance that recombination occurred during formation of its paternal pronucleus.

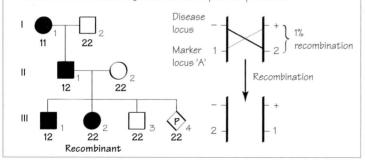

## Linkage analysis in an autosomal recessive disorder

Both parents are heterozygous, having alleles '1' and '2' at a polymorphic marker closely linked to the disease allele. The affected child has inherited allele '1' from both parents so, barring recombination, this is the allele in coupling with the disease allele in both parents. The second child can be offered testing; if she has genotype '11' she is likely to be affected, '22' unaffected and '12' heterozygous.

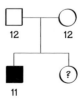

## Overview

If we know the mode of transmission of a monogenic disorder, we can use Mendelian reasoning to predict the probability certain individuals will have affected children (see Chapters 16–20 and 36). Such predictions are, however, never precise. The mapping of the human genome enables a powerful alternative approach based on tracking disease alleles using closely linked polymorphic markers. Use of linkage analysis is limited by the possibility of genetic recombination and the need to collect samples from many family members, but it offers two major advantages: disease genes need not be identified, and we need no molecular understanding of the genes concerned.

## Principle

The linkage approach depends on the concept that genes are organized in the same linear order in (virtually) every person. If a polymorphic locus is revealed to be closely linked to a disease locus, that linkage is true for (almost) all individuals. If a carrier of genetic disease is heterozygous for the polymorphism and the coupling phase of marker and disease alleles can be determined (see Chapter 27), then alleles at the polymorphic locus can be used as markers for the disease.

Intragenic neutral polymorphisms can be used in an adaptation of this approach and in such cases we can assume zero recombination.

### Autosomal dominant traits

In the dominant pedigree (see figure), the affected individual, II-1, is heterozygous for both the disease gene and for alleles '1' and '2' at locus 'A.' The 'A' locus is known from studies in other families to be closely linked to the disease gene, with a 1% rate of recombination between them. Individual II-1 has inherited both the disease allele and allele '1' from his diseased mother, so in this individual marker allele '1' is located on the same chromosome as the disease allele. His partner (II-2) is homozygous for the '2' allele at the marker locus. We can trace the inheritance of the disease allele in their children by determining whether marker allele '1' or '2' was inherited from the father. Child III-1 has inherited allele '1' and is affected, while III-3 has inherited '2' and is unaffected. Child III-2 is an exception as she inherited the '2' allele from her father, yet is affected. This is due to recombination, the probability of which is known from other studies to be 1%. If the unborn child III-4 is a '22' homozygote; the probability he or she will be affected is only 1%, despite the existence of a recombinant sib. If necessary, additional polymorphic flanking markers can be used to confirm such deductions and increase the accuracy of analysis.

### Autosomal recessive traits

Linkage diagnosis can also be performed with recessive traits to follow transmission of alleles from each parent to affected or unaffected children (see figure). In such cases one must use an affected child to infer coupling phases in the parents.

### X-linked traits

The same analysis can be done for X-linked traits, following the inheritance of the two X chromosomes from a heterozygous female. If the grandparental generation is not available for study, one can infer coupling phase from affected children, with the caveat that one or more might be recombinants. This caveat intruduces some uncertainty, and thus decreases analytical power, but it is still better than the estimate of 50% based on the equal probability of inheriting one or the other chromosomal homologue.

Linkage analysis was the mainstay of diagnosis at a time when many disease genes were mapped, but few were cloned. It is less often used today, but is still helpful in instances where the disease gene is mapped but not identified, or where there is a wide diversity of mutations and the gene is large so that molecular analysis is impractical. This is the case currently with the **dystrophin** gene responsible for **Duchenne** and **Becker muscular dystrophies**. The gene has 79 exons and 2/3 of disease alleles have intragenic deletions. The remaining 1/3 have single base pair changes which may be anywhere within the gene. In these, linkage analysis using polymorphic markers remains a powerful approach to carrier testing and prenatal diagnosis (see also Chapters 44, 45).

## Pitfalls in interpretation

There are a number of potential pitfalls in interpretation of linkage-based tests.

**1** The clinical diagnosis in the family must be firmly established, since linkage testing alone will not confirm or refute the original diagnosis.

**2** Different genetic loci are sometimes responsible for clinically indistinguishable disorders. This is the case for **tuberous sclerosis**, where **TSC1** (Chromosome 9) and **TSC2** (Chromosome 16) produce the same condition. Such **genetic heterogeneity** must be taken into account and in some cases may prohibit the use of linkage analysis.

**3** There must be polymorphic markers near the disease locus and these must be heterozygous in an individual heterozygous for the disease allele from whom transmission is being tracked. The high density of the gene map makes this likely but, before diagnostic testing is offered, the family must be studied individually to determine which markers are informative. Specific alleles in coupling with the disease allele will differ between families, though where linkage disequilibrium occurs, one particular allele may be non-randomly associated with disease (see Chapter 27).

**4** Linkage analysis is a family based test and multiple family members must be available and willing to participate in the study. This may present problems with severe recessive disorders if the proband is deceased and their DNA is not available.

**5** Finally, the outcome of a linkage analysis remains only a statistical probability, genetic recombination can always occur and can potentially lead to misdiagnosis.

These reservations over the applicability of linkage analysis must be explained to a family requesting testing and this can be a formidable challenge in counselling.

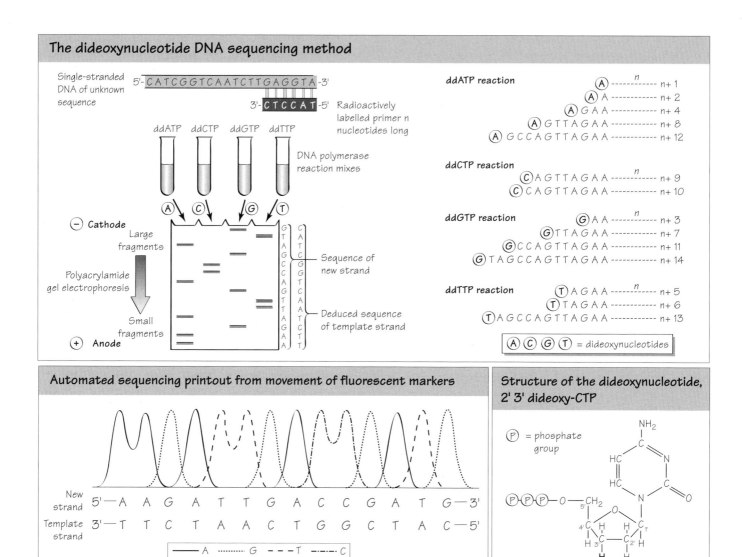

## Overview

A complete description of most mutations requires knowledge of the base sequence of the DNA at the site of error. Currently most DNA sequencing is carried out by the enzymic method of Sanger and co-workers as described here; the end result is a ladder of bands from which the base sequence can be read directly, or a row of peaks on a graph.

## The dideoxy-DNA sequencing method

For this method the DNA to be sequenced is prepared in multiple copies of one 'template' strand. DNA polymerase is then used to synthesize multiple new complementary strands.

The enzymic reaction requires a primer complementary to the 3′ end of the sequence, DNA polymerase, cofactors, etc. and base-specific **dideoxynucleotides** (ddATP, ddTTP, ddCTP and ddGTP), in addition to the normal deoxynucleotide precursors (dATP, etc.). The dideoxynucleotides lack the hydroxyl group present on the 3′ carbon atoms of

deoxynucleotides that in DNA forms the link to the adjacent nucleotide. They are incorporated into growing DNA as normal, but chain extension is blocked beyond them by the lack of the 3′ hydroxyl group. A radioactive or fluorescent label is incorporated either into these ddNTPs or into the primer.

Before the advent of fluorescent technology four parallel base-specific reactions were conducted using a mix of all four normal nucleotide precursors, one with a radioactive label, plus a small proportion of *one* of the four dideoxy- derivatives. If the concentration of the latter is low compared to that of its normal analogue, chain termination occurs randomly at each of the many positions containing that specific base. Each base-specific reaction generates many fragments of different lengths, with variable 3′ termini but a common 5′ end, corresponding to the primer.

The DNA fragments were then separated by electrophoresis through polyacrylamide gel, in which they migrate at speeds inversely proportional to their lengths. Following electrophoresis the gel was dried out and an autoradiographic (or X-ray) film placed in contact with it. After suitable exposure the film was developed to produce a pattern of dark bands. The sequence was then read off by simple inspection of the autoradiograph, providing the 5′-to-3′ sequence of the new strand, complementary to the original template.

This process was automated by attaching four differently coloured fluorescent markers to the four ddNTPs instead of a radioactive label. The DNA synthesis is performed in one vessel and the products run in a single lane of the gel. The migrating bands corresponding to the different DNA fragments are then detected by their fluorescence as they pass through a spot illuminated by a narrow UV light beam. The coloured light signals are monitored electronically and displayed as a row of peaks on a graph.

## Diagnostic applications

DNA sequencing can be used in diagnostic testing, when the aim is to identify *specific* pathogenic mutations. To determine whether a known mutation, or the normal sequence, is present involves sequencing the region of the gene for a short stretch around the mutant site. In an individual heterozygous for a single base substitution two different bases would be found at that site, one representing each DNA strand.

Heterozygous insertions or deletions produce a complex pattern of two superimposed sequences, one mutant and one normal. To elucidate this it may be necessary to clone and sequence the two DNA duplexes separately.

DNA sequencing can also be used to scan large regions of a gene for mutations. This offers the advantage that the specific mutation does not need to be known in advance and can in principle detect a wide variety of types of mutation. However, several precautions must be observed in the interpretation of sequence variants detected in this way. First, not finding a mutation does not necessarily mean no mutation is present:

there may be mutations outside the structural gene, perhaps in regulatory regions. Also, certain types of structural rearrangements, such as deletion of an entire gene, can remain undetected by sequencing. It should also be recognized that not all sequence variants disrupt gene function, as is necessary for it to constitute a pathogenic mutation.

Evidence that a variant is pathogenic might include inference from its likely impact on the gene product; for example, mutations that cause frameshifts are more likely to disrupt function than single base substitutions (see Chapter 30). Demonstration that a mutation is present only in affected individuals and segregates in families together with disease is highly suggestive that that is the gene causing the disorder, or else is in close linkage with it. Another important clue is recapitulation of the mutant phenotype in an animal model based on a known mutation.

Direct sequencing is currently not the method of choice for most diagnostic laboratories, when the goal is to identify the presence of a limited repertoire of mutations. This is the case, for example, with the β-globin mutation responsible for sickle cell anaemia. Since only one mutation is being sought, it is easier and less expensive to use methods of direct mutation analysis, such as PCR followed by restriction enzyme digestion or oligonucleotide hybridization (see Chapters 44 and 45).

Even in analysis of the *CFTR* (cystic fibrosis) gene, where more than 900 mutations have been described, direct sequencing of the entire gene is usually too expensive. Furthermore, sequencing increases sensitivity by only about 10% over analysis of a limited number of relatively common known mutations by techniques like dot-blot oligonucleotide hybridization (Chapter 46).

Direct sequencing is, however, used commonly in the identification of mutations in the breast cancer *BRCA1* and *BRCA2* genes. Here the mutant sites are highly diverse and widely scattered, making it necessary to scan the gene sequences in full.

# 44 Southern blotting

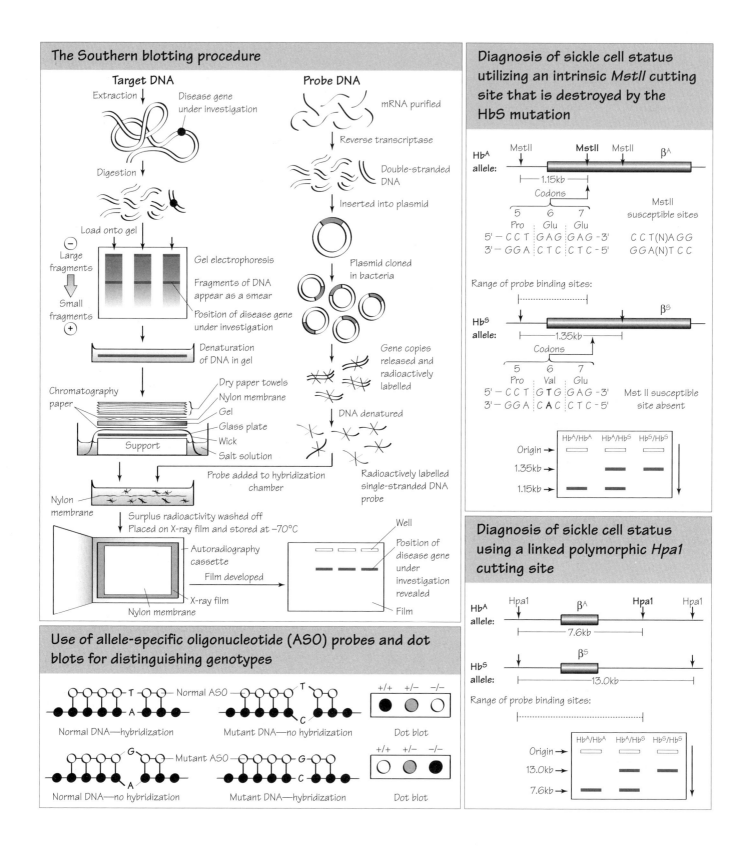

## The Southern blotting procedure

**Target DNA**

Extraction

Disease gene under investigation

Digestion

Load onto gel

(−) Large fragments

Small fragments (+)

Gel electrophoresis

Fragments of DNA appear as a smear

Position of disease gene under investigation

Denaturation of DNA in gel

Chromatography paper — Dry paper towels — Nylon membrane — Gel — Glass plate — Wick — Salt solution

Support

Nylon membrane

Probe added to hybridization chamber

Surplus radioactivity washed off
Placed on X-ray film and stored at −70°C

Autoradiography cassette

Film developed

Nylon membrane

X-ray film

Well

Position of disease gene under investigation revealed

Film

**Probe DNA**

mRNA purified

Reverse transcriptase

Double-stranded DNA

Inserted into plasmid

Plasmid cloned in bacteria

Gene copies released and radioactively labelled

DNA denatured

Radioactively labelled single-stranded DNA probe

## Use of allele-specific oligonucleotide (ASO) probes and dot blots for distinguishing genotypes

T — Normal ASO

Normal DNA—hybridization

G — Mutant ASO

Normal DNA—no hybridization

Mutant DNA—no hybridization

Mutant DNA—hybridization

+/+   +/−   −/−

Dot blot

+/+   +/−   −/−

Dot blot

## Diagnosis of sickle cell status utilizing an intrinsic *MstII* cutting site that is destroyed by the HbS mutation

HbᴬA allele:   MstII   **MstII**   MstII   βᴬ

1.15kb

Codons

MstII susceptible sites

| | 5 | 6 | 7 | |
|---|---|---|---|---|
| | Pro | Glu | Glu | |
| 5' − | C C T | G A G | G A G | -3' |
| 3' − | G G A | C T C | C T C | -5' |

C C T(N)A G G
G G A(N)T C C

Range of probe binding sites:

HbˢS allele:   βˢ

1.35kb

Codons

Mst II susceptible site absent

| | 5 | 6 | 7 | |
|---|---|---|---|---|
| | Pro | Val | Glu | |
| 5' − | C C T | G T G | G A G | -3' |
| 3' − | G G A | C A C | C T C | -5' |

| | Hbᴬ/Hbᴬ | Hbᴬ/Hbˢ | Hbˢ/Hbˢ |
|---|---|---|---|
| Origin → | | | |
| 1.35kb → | | | |
| 1.15kb → | | | |

## Diagnosis of sickle cell status using a linked polymorphic *Hpa1* cutting site

Hbᴬ allele:   Hpa1   βᴬ   **Hpa1**   Hpa1

7.6kb

Hbˢ allele:   βˢ

13.0kb

Range of probe binding sites:

| | Hbᴬ/Hbᴬ | Hbᴬ/Hbˢ | Hbˢ/Hbˢ |
|---|---|---|---|
| Origin → | | | |
| 13.0kb → | | | |
| 7.6kb → | | | |

## Overview

Laboratory confirmation of a clinical diagnosis is often achieved by application of a set of highly specialized molecular techniques collectively known as 'Southern blotting', which allows us to find and examine the one or two DNA fragments of interest in a mixture of millions. Four concepts are necessary to understand the procedure: **DNA probes, restriction endonucleases**, gel electrophoresis and DNA polymorphism.

## DNA probes

A DNA probe is a short section (usually 0.3–5.0 kb) of double-stranded DNA corresponding to part of the locus of interest. It can be prepared, for example, from the **cDNA** (copy DNA) copy of a purified mRNA, generated with the enzyme **reverse transcriptase**, then radioactively labelled and 'denatured' into single strands. Alternatively, cloned segments of genomic DNA can be used.

## Restriction endonucleases and DNA polymorphism

Restriction endonucleases are bacterial enzymes that cut double-stranded DNA at specific sequences. Such sites occur throughout the genome and the sections of DNA that result from enzyme cutting are called **restriction fragments**. Variation in the length of restriction fragments, due to polymorphism at potential cutting sites, is called **restriction fragment length polymorphism** (**RFLP**). These variant cutting sites provide valuable markers for disease genes that can be used in linkage studies (see Chapter 42).

## Gel electrophoresis

A gel is a three-dimensional mesh with pores of different sizes. They are cast as slabs of **agarose** or **polyacrylamide**, with a row of wells at one end for insertion of samples. During electrophoresis the gel is subjected to an electric current, when negatively charged DNA fragments migrate toward the positive terminal or **anode**. The smallest fragments run fastest, with the others behind them in order of size.

## Southern blotting

The usual source of DNA is white blood cells, but for prenatal diagnosis samples may be taken from cultures of chorionic villus, or amniotic fluid cells (see Chapter 41). The DNA is digested with one or more restriction enzymes, inserted into a well of the gel and the electric current applied.

Since the gel is too fragile for manipulation, the electrophoretically fractionated DNA is denatured and transferred to a more durable support, usually a nylon membrane, by the Southern blotting technique (see figure). This in effect produces a print of the DNA array in the gel. The DNA is then bound onto the membrane by exposure to UV light and incubated in a solution containing the denatured radioactive probe. The probe 'hybridizes' with its complementary sequence in the sample. Unbound probe DNA is washed off and the position of the bound radioactivity is located by autoradiography. This involves placing the nylon membrane face down on an X-ray film and storage at –70°C for several hours or days. When the film is developed, black bands appear, indicating the location, and hence the length, of the restriction fragment containing the gene of interest.

Modern approaches use digital systems that detect the radioactivity directly, conferring the advantage of instantaneous results after hybridization. In some instances, non-radioactive labels are used.

## Methodological variants
### Northern blotting

This variant is used to identify mRNA species in a mixture subjected to electrophoresis and probing in a similar way.

### Dot blots and allele-specific oligonucleotides (ASOs)

When both normal and mutant sequences are known very short '**oligonucleotide**' probes can be synthesized biochemically to match each one. These are hybridized to '**dot-blots**' of denatured DNA applied directly to the nylon membrane, allowing rapid identification of homozygotes and heterozygotes, and distinction between alleles.

This approach offers an inexpensive and rapid method of diagnosis, but it is limited by the need for prior knowledge of mutant sequences.

## Diagnostic applications

One application involves selection of a restriction endonuclease for which the recognition site happens to correspond with either the mutant or 'wild type' (i.e. normal) version of the sequence in question. DNA is cut with the enzyme and the resulting fragments are analysed on a Southern blot, using as a probe a DNA sequence near the site of mutation. If the mutation disrupts a normal cutting site, that segment of DNA will remain intact. Presence or absence of the mutation can then be determined by comparing fragment sizes. An example is sickle cell disease (see figure in Chapter 30). In the normal β-globin allele the sixth codon is cut by the enzyme MstII, but the HbS mutation destroys that site and a longer DNA fragment is produced. In most cases polymorphic cutting sites are, however, identified outside the disease gene (see figure).

In most laboratories PCR has replaced Southern analysis for detection of specific alterations in base sequence (see Chapter 45), but it still finds application where larger rearrangements are involved. For example, a large intragenic deletion or inversion may alter the size of a restriction fragment detectable with a particular cDNA probe.

Sometimes deletions are identifiable through Southern analysis by the *reduced intensity* of hybridization of a probe to a restriction fragment. However, this can be difficult to demonstrate as it requires careful attention to quantitative methodology when the blot is prepared. Detection of fragments of altered mobility is simpler and more reliable.

Very long triplet repeat expansions (Chapter 30) cannot be reliably amplified by PCR, but Southern analysis can reveal the expanded allele by its reduced mobility. In Fragile X disease the unexpressed, expanded allele is invariably methylated; differential digestion can therefore be performed with a restriction endonuclease that cleaves only *non-methylated DNA*.

# 45 The polymerase chain reaction

## One cycle of the PCR gene amplification procedure

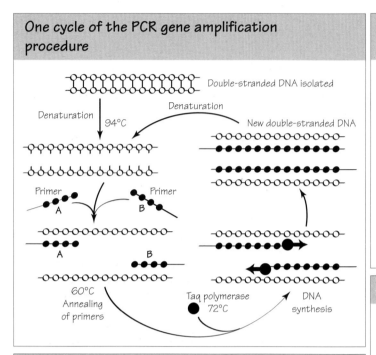

## Use of the ARMS test to distinguish sickle cell and normal β-globin alleles

The normal primer enables amplification of only the normal β-globin allele; the sickle cell primer amplifies only the mutant β-globin DNA

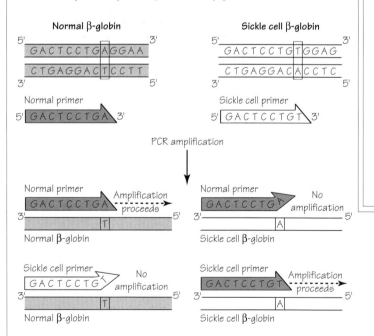

## Use of quantitative PCR for testing a family with Duchenne muscular dystrophy

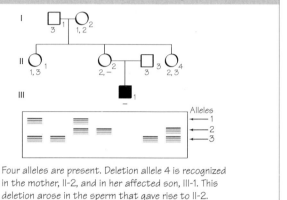

Four alleles are present. Deletion allele 4 is recognized in the mother, II-2, and in her affected son, III-1. This deletion arose in the sperm that gave rise to II-2.

## Use of PCR in testing for Huntington disease

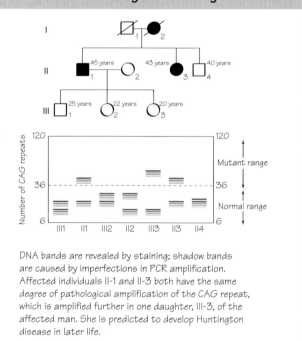

DNA bands are revealed by staining; shadow bands are caused by imperfections in PCR amplification. Affected individuals II-1 and II-3 both have the same degree of pathological amplification of the CAG repeat, which is amplified further in one daughter, III-3, of the affected man. She is predicted to develop Huntington disease in later life.

Sickle cell status revealed by dot-blot hybridization with a labelled β-globin probe

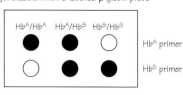

## Overview

The **polymerase chain reaction** (**PCR**) has utterly revolutionized the diagnosis and molecular analysis of genetic disease. Analyses can be performed on samples as minute as a single nucleus obtained from a preimplantation embryo, a mouth wash, hair root, or other source. It is performed in a few hours and is cheaper than any other method. *PCR has therefore become the most widely used method of genetic analysis.*

## The polymerase chain reaction

The reaction uses *Taq* DNA polymerase and operates on single-strand DNA, replacing the missing strand in much the same way as in DNA replication (see Chapter 5). *Taq* polymerase is isolated from *Thermus aquaticus*, a hot spring bacterium, and can withstand temperatures up to 95°C. It requires a start point of duplex DNA, which is provided by single-strand **primers** annealed one at each end of the sequence to be duplicated.

To carry out the reaction the DNA sample is first heated to 94°C to 'melt' the hydrogen bonds joining the two polynucleotide strands. The temperature is reduced to ~60° and the short oligonucleotide primers are added. These are usually 15–30 nucleotides long and designed to match and anneal to complementary conserved stretches flanking the chosen sequence. In the third step, carried out at 72°, the polymerase moves down the DNA strand, away from the primers and synthesizes a complementary strand, so recreating a double-stranded molecule.

This set of three steps can be considered as one 'cycle', which is repeated by careful temperature control in the presence of excess primers. Each cycle takes only a few minutes and the amount of DNA doubles every time. After 30 cycles over 100 000 000 copies of the original sequence are created. The process is normally performed automatically in a programmed thermocycler.

PCR can also be used to amplify RNA sequences, if they are first copied into cDNA replicates by means of reverse transcriptase.

## Comparative advantages of PCR

1 **Sensitivity**: PCR is applicable to single-genome quantities of DNA.
2 **Speed**: the procedure is very fast (3–48 h).
3 **Safety**: no radioactivity is involved.
4 **Molecular product**: the product is suitable for further analysis by established molecular techniques.
5 **Resolution**: the process can be applied to even badly degraded DNA.

## Disadvantages of PCR

1 **Size of template**: long sequences cannot be amplified.
2 **Prior knowledge**: the base sequences of flanking regions must be known.
3 **Contamination**: absolute purity of sample is essential.
4 **Infidelity of replication**: there is no 'proof-reading', or error correction, so that mutations that occasionally arise during the process are also propagated.

## Diagnostic applications

The value of PCR in diagnosis lies in its ability to provide large quantities of specific gene sequences that can be subjected to further analysis. Primers are used that flank one specific region of a gene, or alternatively multiple regions such as several exons. Applications include the following:

1 **Diagnosis of triplet repeat disorders** (e.g. DMD and Huntington disease; see figure and Chapters 30 and 44).
2 **Direct sequencing** of the gene(s) (see Chapter 43).
3 **Restriction endonuclease digestion**. This approach can be applied when a *specific* mutation is being sought. An endonuclease is chosen that has a recognition sequence spanning the mutant site (see Chapter 44). The enzyme will then either cut or not cut the DNA, depending on whether the mutation is present. Analysis of fragment sizes by agarose gel electrophoresis then indicates the genotype.
4 **Single strand conformation polymorphism** (**SSCP**). In this method PCR amplified DNA is denatured and electrophoresed without renaturation, when mutant strands are detectable by their abnormal speeds of migration.
5 **Allele specific oligonucleotide** (**ASO**) **binding**. This method, described in Chapter 44, is commonly used where analysis involves detection of a single mutation (e.g. sickle cell disease) or a limited range of *common* disease alleles (e.g. cystic fibrosis).
6 **The amplification refractory mutation system** (**ARMS**) depends on specificity of binding of PCR primers to template DNA (see figure). A primer is designed with a 3′ end corresponding to either a mutant, or the wild type sequence. The primer will bind only with its exact complement, so a wild type primer permits amplification of only wild type DNA, mutant primer only mutant DNA. Two separate PCR reactions, with either mutant or wild type primer, together with another primer elsewhere in the gene, can be used to determine heterozygosity or homozygosity of either sequence. This approach also has been used to identify CFTR mutations.
7 **Quantitative PCR**. PCR is used routinely for quantitative detection of deletions in the dystrophin gene responsible for **Duchenne muscular dystrophy**. Since this gene is on the X chromosome, affected males entirely lack certain exons. PCR primers that flank these exons yield no DNA product, making them identifiable by default, but since the gene is very large it is necessary to check many exons. A multiplex mix of primers, each responsible for one region, enables this to be done in a single reaction. The various products are then revealed by agarose gel electrophoresis followed by DNA staining. Deletion of an exon is indicated by one or more missing bands.

Quantitative detection of heterozygous deletions, as with female carriers of muscular dystrophy, is more difficult. Quantification of PCR products is possible but requires special equipment and considerable analytical care. It is more practicable to use FISH applied to a chromosome spread (see Chapter 38) once the deletion has been established in the proband and an appropriate DNA probe prepared.
8 **DNA profiling**. See Chapter 46.

## 46 DNA profiling

### Use of minisatellite polymorphism for DNA profiling

The structure of two minisatellite alleles. Probe 1 is based on the core sequence repeat and Probe 2 on a unique flanking sequence. Cutting sites for restriction endonucleases, *Eco R1* and *Bam H1*, are shown

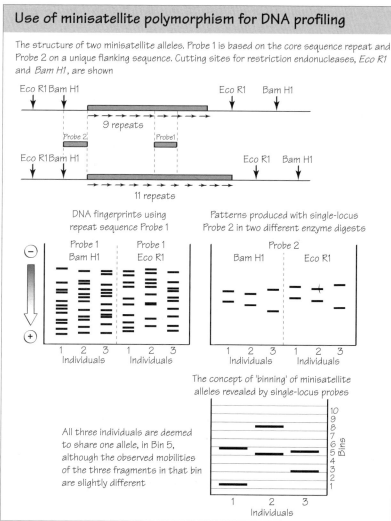

9 repeats

11 repeats

DNA fingerprints using repeat sequence Probe 1

Patterns produced with single-locus Probe 2 in two different enzyme digests

The concept of 'binning' of minisatellite alleles revealed by single-locus probes

All three individuals are deemed to share one allele, in Bin 5, although the observed mobilities of the three fragments in that bin are slightly different

### Microsatellite repeat polymorphisms amplified by PCR

A range of alleles defined by numbers of repeats of the core sequence /TACT/

Primer 1

$(TACT)_{10}$ A
$(TACT)_{11}$ B
$(TACT)_{12}$ C
$(TACT)_{13}$ D
$(TACT)_{14}$ E
$(TACT)_{15}$ F

Primer 2

Mobility patterns of alleles after electrophoresis, alongside a reference standard

Repeat number

Ref. B/D A/F E/D B/E A/A C/F E/E Ref.

Genotype of individuals

### Practical applications of DNA fingerprinting

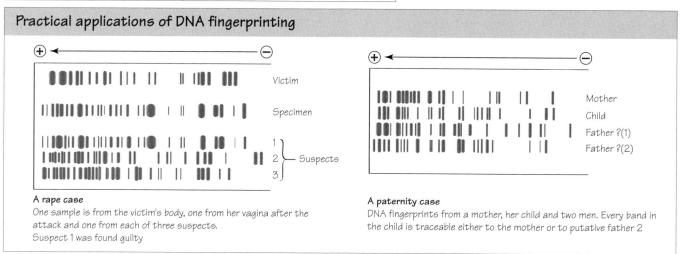

Victim
Specimen
1
2  }  Suspects
3

**A rape case**
One sample is from the victim's body, one from her vagina after the attack and one from each of three suspects.
Suspect 1 was found guilty

Mother
Child
Father ?(1)
Father ?(2)

**A paternity case**
DNA fingerprints from a mother, her child and two men. Every band in the child is traceable either to the mother or to putative father 2

## Overview

**DNA profiling** is the characterization of an individual genome by DNA analysis. It includes **DNA fingerprinting**, use of **single locus probes**, microsatellite, Y-chromosome, mitochondrial and ethnic polymorphisms. It is of enormous value for identifying the father in paternity disputes, for confirming family membership in immigration cases and for identifying the perpetrators and victims of crime from traces of biological material.

As explained in Chapter 4, our genomes contain a large quantity of highly repetitive DNA called '**microsatellite DNA**', when the sequence is short (1–4 bp), and '**minisatellite DNA**', when the sequence is longer (5–64 bp). Microsatellite DNA is scattered throughout the chromosomes and provides useful markers for disease genes (see Chapter 42). Minisatellite DNA is concentrated near the centromeres and telomeres and is particularly valuable for DNA profiling, but both are exploited in this respect.

## Application of Southern blotting
### DNA fingerprinting with minisatellite markers

The Southern blotting approach to DNA analysis (see Chapter 46) depends on the creation of **RFLPs** due to polymorphism at restriction endonuclease cutting sites. DNA fingerprinting also depends on fragment length polymorphism, but due to variation instead in the number of repetitious sequences between cutting sites. These are known as **variable number tandem repeats** (**VNTRs**).

The first probe used in fingerprinting was directed against the repeated minisatellite **core sequence /GGGCAGGAXG/**, where X is any nucleotide. Tandem repeats of two to several hundred copies of this sequence are present in the human genome at over 1000 sites, although only 8–17 are of practical value in fingerprinting.

If a sample of human DNA is digested with a restriction enzyme for which there are many cutting sites (a '**frequent cutter**'), multiple fragments are produced of many sizes and of great variation between individuals. Those fragments that contain repeats of the core sequence can be visualized on Southern blots by the core sequence probe, as a ladder of bands (see figure). The chances of any two unrelated individuals having the same pattern are estimated at less than $1/10^{11}$. The only exceptions are members of genetic clones, such as MZ twins. These patterns are known as '**DNA fingerprints**' (see figure).

The statistical evaluation of multilocus fingerprint evidence in forensic casework rests on the proportion ($x$) of bands which on average are shared by unrelated people. '$x$' is estimated as 0.14 for both the most commonly used probes, irrespective of ethnicity. A conservative estimate of 0.25 is normally used to prevent over-interpretation and to allow for possible relationship between suspect and guilty party.

Assuming statistical independence of (i.e. no linkage between) all bands then the chance that $n$ bands in individual A are matched by bands of precisely similar electrophoretic mobility in B is $x$ to the power $n$ ($x^n$).

In paternity disputes germline mutation can lead to invalid exclusion of a putative father. In fact 27% of offspring show one band not present in either parent, 1.2% show two and an estimated <0.3% show three new bands.

Repetitious regions containing multiples of other core sequences can be exploited to produce different fingerprints, using the same enzyme digest and appropriate probes. Alternatively, the same DNA sample can be digested with a different restriction enzyme and examined with the same probe or others.

## Use of single-locus probes

If a fingerprinting blot is examined with a probe complementary to a sequence *flanking* one hypervariable region a much simplified pattern is revealed, derived from just that one locus (see figure). Each such probe should reveal a maximum of two bands in any person, representing the two alleles and on average 70% of people are heterozygous at any such locus.

Statistical proof of identity requires examination of 4–10 such loci and if the population frequency of each 'allele' is known, it is possible to make exact calculations of probability. However, exact numbers of repeats are not always known and fragment band positions do not always correspond precisely. So for statistical purposes the DNA track is divided into a number of 'bins' and bands are deemed to match if they fall within the same bin. Although 'binning' introduces inaccuracies it is necessary to estimate the population frequencies of fragments of specific lengths. This is always done conservatively, so that the statistical weight of evidence is biased in favour of the defendant. Appropriate ethnic databases also have to be set up and when applying Hardy–Weinberg reasoning (see Chapter 26) due allowance must be made for possible population stratification based on, for example, ethnicity, religion or class.

## Application of PCR

PCR amplification (see Chapter 45) dramatically increases the potential range of forensic analysis to minute samples and degraded material. It can be applied to minisatellite polymorphisms by use of primers based on unique sequences flanking the tandem repeat arrays. However, the introduction of PCR also brings formidable problems of sample contamination (see Chapter 45).

The most common microsatellites are runs of A, AC or AG. In PCR applications they have the advantage over minisatellites in that discrete alleles can be defined unambiguously by the precise number of repeats, calibrated by the mobility of standards. This avoids the requirement for some aspects of statistical proof and makes it easier to relate experimental findings to allele frequencies.

Y-chromosome and mitochondrial DNA polymorphisms are especially useful in some circumstances because of their sex-specific modes of transmission (Chapter 20).

Human DNA is distinguishable from non-human by testing for hybridization with a probe directed at the human-specific *Alu* repeat. In theory at least, probes could also be designed to detect population-specific polymorphisms that might indicate the ethnic origin of an individual.

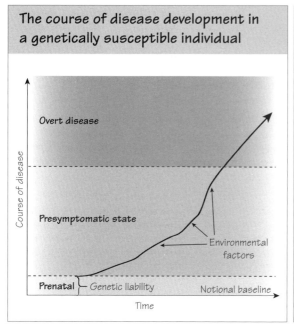

The course of disease development in a genetically susceptible individual

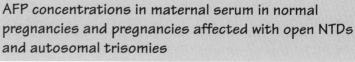

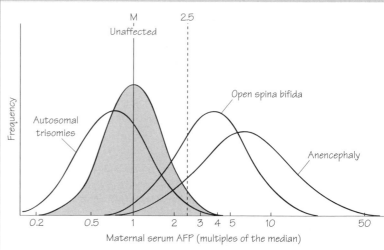

AFP concentrations in maternal serum in normal pregnancies and pregnancies affected with open NTDs and autosomal trisomies

## Overview

The genes each of us inherits contribute some degree of liability toward many disorders. In the case of fully penetrant monogenic diseases, one or a pair of defective alleles alone confers sufficient liability to cause disease. In other instances genetic liability is expressed merely as a susceptibility, and manifestation of disease requires the passage of time and/or accumulation of specific environmental exposures (see figure). **Preventive genetics** is based on testing for factors that contribute to genetic liability. This identifies persons at risk, enabling them to be educated about individually hazardous environmental factors and providing opportunities for modification of lifestyles. In some cases proactive treatment can be offered to reduce risks, or surveillance to ensure early diagnosis and the prompt institution of therapy.

There are three classes of heterozygous carrier for which **population screening** might be appropriate:

1 autosomal recessive diseases of high incidence;
2 relatively common X-linked disorders;
3 autosomal dominant disorders of late onset.

A genetic disease is suitable for population screening if it is clearly defined, of appreciable frequency and early diagnosis is advantageous. The test should be easily performed, be non-invasive and yield few false positives or false negatives. Screening should be widely available, morally acceptable and preferably show a net cost benefit. Appropriate information and counselling should also be available.

## Prenatal screening

### Neural tube defects

Pregnancies with open neural tube defects (NTD) are detectable at 16 weeks by assay of alpha-fetoprotein (AFP) concentration in amniotic fluid and in many cases also in maternal serum. However, in maternal serum there is overlap between unaffected and NTD pregnancies, so an arbitrary concentration is observed below which no further action is taken. A cut-off at 2.5 multiples of the normal median identifies >90% of fetuses with anencephaly and ~80% of those with open NTDs (see figure).

Over 20 years maternal serum screening, with dietary improvements and preconceptional folic acid supplementation have yielded a 25-fold decrease in NTDs in England and Wales.

### Down syndrome

The combination of maternal age and abnormal concentrations of four biochemicals in a mother's serum can identify most pregnancies with Down syndrome (see Chapter 41). At 16 weeks, concentrations of AFP and **unconjugated oestriol** tend to be reduced in the blood of women pregnant with babies with Down syndrome, whereas that of **human chorionic gonadotrophin (hCG)** is raised. The 'triple test' combining the three identifies 60% of pregnancies with Down syndrome. Inclusion of **inhibin A**, increased in pregnancies with Down syndrome, raises this to 75%. Incorporation of the ultrasonographic observation of **increased fetal nuchal transparency** (abnormal accumulation of fluid behind the baby's neck) at 12 weeks, with confirmation by cytogenetic testing, detects 80% of babies with Down syndrome.

### Neonatal screening

If neonatal screening is to be undertaken the consultative follow-up should be prompt and involve definitive diagnosis, prompt initiation of management and appropriate genetic counselling.

**Phenylketonuria**, **galactosaemia** and **congenital hypothyroidism** all cause mental disability, but can be screened for in newborns and prophylactic regimes imposed. Screening for phenylketonuria is routine in most developed countries, galactosaemia screening is less common. Congenital hypothyroidism is not usually genetic, but screening is routine in many countries.

The test for galactosaemia is similar to the Guthrie test for PKU (see Chapter 39), with confirmation by enzyme assay. Screening for hypothyroidism involves assay of thyroxine and thyroid stimulating hormone.

## Cystic fibrosis
Currently neonatal diagnosis of cystic fibrosis is based on immunological quantification of trypsin in the blood, supplemented by DNA analysis (see Chapter 45). Up to 80% of heterozygotes are detected by tests for the $\Delta$F508 allele and a further 10% by multiplex tests for several rarer alleles, depending on ethnicity.

## Sickle cell disease
Several techniques have been used for diagnosis of sickle cell anaemia, including electrophoresis of haemoglobin, demonstration of red cell sickling at low oxygen tensions and a range of DNA tests (see Chapters 44 and 45).

## Thalassaemia
Populations for which thalassaemia carrier screening programmes might prove, or have proved, advantageous include China and East Asia (for alpha-thalassaemia), the Indian subcontinent and Mediterranean countries (for beta-thalassaemia). In Cyprus, screening has led to a 95% decline in babies with beta-thalassaemia in 10 years.

**Table 47.1** Estimated new genetic abnormalities in 1 million live births in a population exposed to low-dose radiation equivalent to 1 rad of X-rays.*

| Category | Number of cases |
| --- | --- |
| Aberrant chromosomes | 38 |
| Autosomal dominant and X-linked | 20 |
| Recessive lesions | 30 |
| Multifactorial diseases | 5 |

*Numbers based on atomic bomb survival statistics and animal experiments.

## Tay–Sachs disease
Carrier screening followed by prenatal diagnosis and termination has reduced Tay–Sachs disease by 95% among American Ashkenazi Jews.

## Screening for adult-onset disease
Late-onset diseases for which screening may be advised include **Huntington disease**, **myotonic dystrophy**, **retinitis pigmentosa** and **spinal cerebellar ataxia**. Early diagnosis of these can allow psychological, emotional and financial preparation. Predictive testing for inherited cancer predisposition, such as **familial adenomatous polyposis** and **breast/ovarian cancer** can ensure inclusion in clinical surveillance programmes and the possibility of prophylactic surgery.

## Occupational screening
In the workplace genetic screening is done to monitor genetic damage due to exposure to ionizing radiation (see Chapter 29 and Table 47.1) or for susceptibility to specific environmental chemicals. Around 50 genetic traits are related to specific environmental agents (Table 47.2). These include **G6PD deficiency**, for which oxidants such as ozone and nitrogen dioxide are contra-indicated and the **sickle cell trait**, carriers of which are highly susceptible to carbon monoxide and cyanide.

## Genetic registers
Genetic registers are registers of local families with genetic disease. Their primary purpose is to maintain two-way contact between the clinical genetics unit and relevant family members. This ensures families do not feel excluded from a source of support and allows investigation to be offered as appropriate.

They are most valuable for relatively common conditions of late onset, with potentially serious effects that are amenable to prevention or treatment.

## Negative implications of screening programs
Negative implications can include:
1 inaccuracy of test results;
2 invasion of privacy;
3 stigmatization;
4 implied compulsion;
5 the 'right to not know' about one's genetic deficiencies;
6 leakage of confidential data.

**Table 47.2** Genetic conditions that create health risks with specific environmental agents.

| Genetic susceptibility | Environmental agent | Resultant condition |
| --- | --- | --- |
| G6PD deficiency | Fava beans, mothballs, ozone, nitrogen dioxide | Haemolytic crisis |
| Sickle cell trait | Cyanide, carbon monoxide | Haemolytic crisis |
| Hypercholesterolaemia | Saturated fats | Atherosclerosis |
| Gluten sensitivity | Wheat protein | Coeliac disease |
| Defective Na/K pump | Common salt | Hypertension |
| Lactose intolerance | Milk sugar | Colic and diarrhoea |
| Deficient ADH | Alcohol | Alcoholism |
| Deficient ALDH | Alcohol | Flushing response |
| Hyperoxaluria | Oxalates (e.g. in spinach) | Kidney stones |
| Haemochromatosis | Iron food supplement | Iron overload |
| $\alpha$1-antitrypsin deficiency | Tobacco smoke | Emphysema |
| Atopic diathesis | Pollen | Hay fever |

# 48 The management of genetic disease

## Control points for potential management of genetic disease

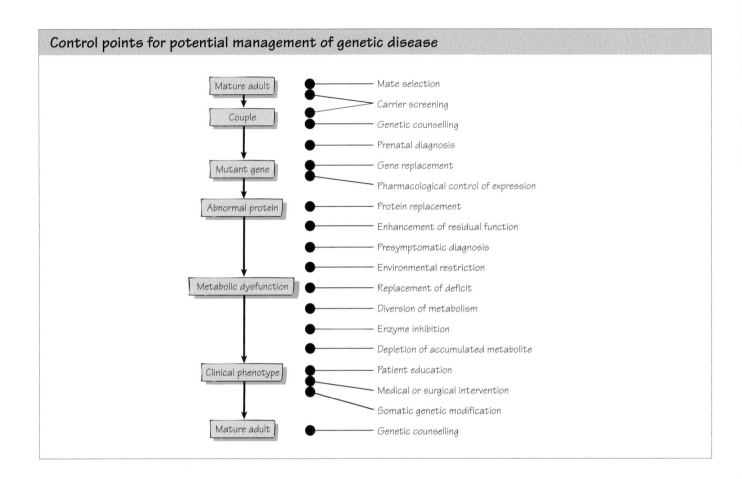

| | |
|---|---|
| Mature adult | Mate selection |
| | Carrier screening |
| Couple | Genetic counselling |
| | Prenatal diagnosis |
| Mutant gene | Gene replacement |
| | Pharmacological control of expression |
| Abnormal protein | Protein replacement |
| | Enhancement of residual function |
| | Presymptomatic diagnosis |
| | Environmental restriction |
| Metabolic dysfunction | Replacement of deficit |
| | Diversion of metabolism |
| | Enzyme inhibition |
| | Depletion of accumulated metabolite |
| Clinical phenotype | Patient education |
| | Medical or surgical intervention |
| | Somatic genetic modification |
| Mature adult | Genetic counselling |

## Overview

Genetic disease can potentially be avoided altogether or ameliorated at several points during a generation, or during expression of the gene (see Chapter 47). For example, in some orthodox Jewish groups partnerships are arranged by matchmakers who consider, among other things, carrier status for Tay–Sachs disease. Correction of overt genetic defects can involve surgery, physiological adjustment or the switching on of genes that are not normally expressed.

With the near completion of the Human Genome Project (see Chapter 28) technologies are being developed aimed at screening DNA samples for possibly hundreds of thousands of **single nucleotide polymorphisms (SNPs)** in one operation. The most promising approaches involve spotting multitudes of detector clones onto glass wafers or 'chips' by application of semiconductor manufacturing techniques. These chips are designed to be screened robotically allowing rapid selection of patients for personalized management.

Genetics is also providing new insights into pathogenesis, enabling development of new pharmacological therapies and inspiring entirely novel approaches such as '**gene therapy**', involving control, replacement or modification of defective genes.

## Correction of gross phenotype

Surgical correction of cleft lip and palate, cleft palate, pyloric stenosis and congenital heart defects accounts for the treatment of 20–30% of all infants with major genetically determined disorders.

## Correction of metabolic dysfunction

**1 Environmental restriction**. This includes avoidance of tobacco smoke by those with emphysema due to **α1-antitrypsin deficiency**, of skin diving and high altitude flying by sickle cell heterozygotes, of sunlight by patients with albinism, porphyria and xeroderma pigmentosa and of X-rays by those with the chromosome breakage syndromes.

A diet low in phenylalanine is most effective in ensuring normal brain development in children with phenylketonuria (see Chapter 42), although this must be administered immediately after birth and maintained into early adulthood. Similar diets adopted by female homozygotes before and during pregnancy can prevent abnormal development of their (heterozygous) babies.

The early exclusion of galactose and lactose prevents serious complications in babies homozygous for galactosaemia.

**2 Replacement of deficit.** Examples are provision of thyroid hormone for hypothyroidism, Factor VIII for haemophilia, and vitamin D for dark-skinned children in Northern climates. Bone marrow transplantation is effective for correction of inherited immune defects such as **SCID** (see Chapter 33).

**3 Diversion of metabolism.** This includes stimulation of alternative pathways, as in correction of **urea cycle** disorders, and enhancement of expression of the normal allele in heterozygotes for **familial hypercholesterolaemia**.

**4 Enzyme inhibition.** Competitive inhibition of rate-controlling enzymes has proved effective, e.g. in familial hypercholesterolaemia.

**5 Enhancement of enzyme function.** This can sometimes be achieved by administration of a cofactor, e.g. vitamin B6 for **homocystinuria**.

**6 Depletion of accumulated metabolite.** An example is renal dialysis for obviating the complications of defective kidney function.

## Modulation of gene expression

Examples are administration of hydroxyurea to **sickle cell** patients to restimulate synthesis of fetal haemoglobin ($\alpha 2, \gamma 2$) and the (so far, experimental) transcription of 'antisense' oligonucleotides to neutralize newly synthesized mRNA by hybridization in cancer cells.

## Gene replacement

The ultimate approach to therapy of genetic disorders is replacement of the defective gene, but such attempts have met with mixed success. For example, inhalation of disabled cold virus (**adenovirus**) carrying a copy of the normal CFTR allele has proved only temporarily effective in the treatment of cystic fibrosis. A successful example is replacement of the **adenosine deaminase** gene in bone marrow cells of children with **SCID** (see above and Chapter 33).

The principle of gene therapy is that an extrinsic gene is introduced into a cell and expressed either as a free-standing gene or, after integration, into a chromosome and transmission at cell division.

Prerequisites are:

**1** the gene concerned and its control elements must be fully characterized and cloned;

**2** accessible target cells must be identified that have a reasonable productive life span;

**3** the chosen vector system must be efficient and safe.

A variety of methods have been used to introduce genes into cells, including incubation with 'naked' DNA or DNA enclosed within artificial lipoprotein vesicles called **liposomes**. Other approaches utilize **retroviruses**, which have their own means for introducing genes into chromosomes.

In spite of encouraging results, major challenges remain. These include how to introduce the therapeutic gene into the *correct* target cells and obtain *physiologically meaningful* levels of expression. Some target cells, especially those in the central nervous system, are not readily accessible. Even if they can be reached by vectors, there is no certainty the introduced genes will be expressed at appropriate levels or be subject to normal regulation. There is also concern that chromosomal integration of vectors may disrupt other genes, causing side-effects as bad or even worse than the original disease.

## Pharmacogenomics

Genetic testing is vital for characterizing metabolic peculiarities and for prescribing drug dosages compatible with individual metabolic rates. But whether or not predictive testing becomes widely established, elucidation of the genetic components of disease is suggesting new approaches to therapy. New drugs are already being developed that target specific proteins involved in disease processes revealed through genetic studies. An example is the drug *Gleevac*, that blocks binding of ATP by the fusion protein formed from the *BCR/abl* gene rearrangement in CML (see Chapter 32). This causes significant tumour shrinkage, although relapses occur as tumour cells acquire resistance.

Genes have also been introduced into cancer cells in the hope of stimulating an immune response, while another anticancer measure involves injecting a *Herpes* virus-based vector expressing thymidine kinase directly into brain tumours, making their cells hypersensitive to the normally non-toxic anti-*Herpes* drug, *Ganciclovir*.

# Glossary

**A**: adenine; blood group A

**AB**: blood group AB

**AD**: autosomal dominant

**AFP**: alpha-fetoprotein

**AR**: autosomal recessive

**adenocarcinoma**: malignant tumour of glandular tissue

**adenoma**: non-malignant tumour of glandular tissue

**allele frequency**: 'gene frequency'; the number of genetic loci at which a particular allele is found, divided by the number of alleles at that locus in the population

*Alu* **repeat**: the most abundant repeat sequence in the human genome, found only in primates

**anticipation**: onset of genetic disease at younger ages in later generations or with increasing severity in each generation

**anticodon**: sequence of three bases within tRNA that is the base pair rule complement to a specific triplet codon and is utilized as such in the translation of mRNA into polypeptide

**anti-sense strand**: template strand of DNA

**apoptosis**: programmed cell death

**ascertainment**: recognition of individuals with a specified phenotype

**assortative mating**: mate selection on the basis of specific characters

**ATP**: adenosine triphosphate

**B**: blood group B

**balanced polymorphism**: genetic polymorphism maintained in a population by opposing selective forces

**BCL**: bilateral cleft lip

*BCR*: break point cluster region of Chromosome 22 involved in the translocation seen in most cases of CML

**benign tumour**: abnormal, compact mass of cells that does not endanger life

**bivalent**: homologous pair of chromosomes while pairing during meiosis

**bp**: base pair

**C**: cytosine; haploid number of single-strand chromosomes; number of concordant twin pairs

**2C**: diploid number of single-strand chromosomes

**cancer**: breakdown in homeostatic control of cell growth leading to metastasis

**candidate gene**: genetic locus plausibly involved in causing disease

**carcinoma**: malignant tumour of the skin or epithelial mucus membrane

**cDNA**: DNA copy of a specific mRNA synthesized by reverse transcriptase

**cellular oncogene**: proto-oncogene

**centimorgan**: genetic map distance between two loci that are segregated on average in 1% of meioses

**Central Dogma**: concept that genetic information is transferred in the cell in the direction DNA→RNA→protein

*CFTR*: cystic fibrosis transmembrane regulator; the cystic fibrosis gene

**chiasma**: connection between the chromatids of homologous chromosomes where crossing over is occurring at meiosis

**chromatid**: one of the two strands which result from duplication of a chromosome, found during prophase and metaphase of mitosis and meiosis. Each chromatid contains a single, very long molecule of DNA. They separate at anaphase and are then known as daughter chromosomes

**chromatin**: the material components of chromosomes

**chromosome abnormality**: phenotypically significant change in chromosome number or structure

*cis* **conformation**: presence of alleles of different genes on the same strand of DNA, c.f. *trans*

**clone**: two or more individuals derived from one genome.

**CL+/-P**: cleft lip with or without cleft palate

**CML**: chronic myelogenous leukaemia

**CNS**: central nervous system

**codominance**: expression of both alleles in a heterozygote

**codon**: a sequence of three bases within a gene, that corresponds to a specific amino acid in the corresponding polypeptide

**concordance**: degree to which relatives, especially twins, share a particular trait

**consultand**: individual who approached the clinician for genetic advice.

**consanguinuity**: genetic relationship

**continuous variation**: variation in a character which forms a continuous series from one extreme to the other

**coupling**: *cis* conformation

**D**: number of discordant twin pairs

**deletion**: loss of some or all of a gene or chromosome

**ΔF508**: the most common mutation causative of cystic fibrosis

*der*: derivative chromosome

**diploid**: having twice the haploid content of chromosomes, i.e. the normal full complement

**discontinuous variation**: the existence of two or more non-overlapping classes with respect to a particular character

**DNA**: deoxyribonucleic acid

**DNA binding protein**: protein which affects gene activity by becoming attached to the DNA

**DNA fingerprint**: pattern of hypervariable minisatellite DNA repeats unique to each individual

**DNA hybridization**: reassembly of complemetary pairs of DNA single strands into a double-strand by base pairing

**DNA probe**: small fragment of single-strand DNA with the same sequence of nucleotides as the section of native human DNA of interest, labelled with a radioactive or fluorescent tag

**DNA renaturation**: DNA hybridization

**dominant**: an allele is said to be dominant over an alternative allele at the same locus when it, rather than the alternative allele, is expressed in a heterozygote

**DOPA**: dihydroxyphenylalanine

**dot blot**: DNA, usually amplified by PCR, applied directly to a membrane without electrophoresis

**dynamic mutation**: transient or progressive change in the DNA that affects its coding properties or degree of expression

**DZ**: dizygotic, arising from two zygotes

**empiric risk**: observed frequency of disease in a given situation

**ER**: endoplasmic reticulum

**expressivity**: degree to which an allele is expressed in an individual

**FAP(C)**: familial adenomatous polyposis (coli)

**fixation**: elimination of alternative alleles in a population

**frameshift mutation**: mutation involving loss or gain of nucleotides of a number not divisible by three, so that the translational reading frame is put out of register

**G**: guanine

**G0, G1, G2**: phases of the mitotic cycle

**G-bands**: pattern of AT-rich dark bands produced in chromosomes by special treatment followed by Giemsa staining

**gene**: the basic unit of inheritance

**gene expression**: creation of a phenotypic character corresponding to a gene. It is frequently (but erroneously) considered as synonymous with transcription

**gene flow**: geographical movement of alleles by migration

**gene frequency**: see 'allele frequency'

**gene map**: representation of the relative positions of the genes in the genome

**gene therapy**: therapeutic correction of an inherited defect at the level of the gene

**genetic association**: occurrence of a specific allele with a specific phenotype at frequency greater than expected by chance

**genetic code**: set of correpondences between triplet codons of bases in mRNA and amino acids in polypeptides

**genetic drift**: non-selective change in allele frequency

**genetic heterogeneity**: similar genetic condition caused by different genes

**genome**: genetic content of a haploid cell; the genetic makeup of a species

**genotype**: genetic constitution of an individual

**germline mutation**: mutation that can be transmitted to offspring

**G6PD**: glucose-6-phosphate dehydrogenase

**haploid**: possessing only one copy of the genetic material, as in a sperm or ovum

**haplotype**: set of alleles of linked genes that tend to be inherited together

**HbA**: normal allele for β-globin

**HbS**: sickle cell allele of β-globin

**heritability**: the fraction of phenotypic variation that can be ascribed to genotypic variation

**heterozygote**: individual with dissimilar alleles of a particular gene

**hnRNA**: heterogeneous nuclear RNA

**homozygote**: individual with similar alleles of a particular gene

**human genome**: theoretical concept that includes the genomes of all normal human beings, as well as the idea of an 'average' or typical genome for a human

**Human Genome Project**: ongoing project to map and sequence the entire human genome.

**hypervariable DNA**: fraction of non-coding DNA consisting of repetitive sequences that shows a great deal of variation in repeat number between individuals

**Ig**: immunoglobulin

**imprinting**: acquisition by a gene of a semi-permanent modification that affects its expression. Imprinting can be changed in a subsequent generation

**inbreeding**: breeding between individuals who share one or more common ancestors

**inbreeding depression**: reduction in fitness caused by homozygosity of certain alleles due to inbreeding

**incest**: sexual intercourse between close relatives, usually those sharing 25% or more of their genetic material

**index case**: proband

**karyotype**: a formula that describes the somatic chromosome complement of an individual or a photomicrograph of his/her metaphase chromosomes arranged in standard order

**kb**: kilobase (1000 bases)

**liability**: inherited predisposition

**linked**: of genes, close together on the same chromosome

**linkage disequilibrium**: co-occurrence of closely linked alleles more frequently than expected by chance

**linkage phase**: situation of alternative pairs of alleles with respect to one another on homologous chromosomes

**location score**: the equivalent in multilocus mapping of lod scores in two-point mapping

**lod**: 'Log of the odds'; the logarithm ($\log_{10}$) of the ratio of the probability that a certain combination of phenotypes arose as a result of genetic linkage (of a specified degree) to the probability that it arose merely by chance

**lod score**: the total value of the combined lods for a family or group of families calculated at the most probable degree of linkage

**M**: monosomy; mitotic phase of the cell cycle

**M1, M2**: first, second divisions of meiosis

**malignancy**: ability of cells to sustain proliferation and invade other tissues

**malignant tumour**: tumour with the capacity for unrestrained growth and shedding of invasive cells

**Mb**: megabase (1000,000 bases)

**Mendel's laws**: set of rules governing inheritance of single-gene features discovered by Gregor Mendel, sometimes presented as the 'Law of Segregation of Genetic Factors' and the 'Law of Independent Assortment of Genetic Factors'

**metaphase plate**: arrangement of chromosomes that forms across the main axis of the spindle apparatus at metaphase

**metastasis**: transfer of cancer cells about the body

**MHC**: major histocompatibility complex

**microsatellite DNA**: category of repetitive DNA with tandem repeats of a very short sequence, e.g. 1-4 base pairs

**minisatellite DNA**: category of repetitive DNA with tandem repeats of a sequence of intermediate length, e.g. 10-15 base pairs

**MIS**: Mullerian inhibiting substance

**mitosis-suppressor gene**: tumour suppressor gene; the normal allele of such a gene suppresses cell division, usually at the transition from G1 to S-, or G2 to M-phase of the mitotic cycle

**monosomy**: presence of only one copy of a chromosome

**mosaic**: existence in the body of more than one population of genetically distinct cells

**mRNA**: messenger RNA

**multifactorial trait**: character that results from the joint action of several factors, including genes and environmental influences

**multipoint map**: gene map based on several reference loci

**mutagen**: environmental agent capable of causing damage to DNA

**mutator gene**: faulty DNA repair gene

**mutation**: process by which a gene undergoes a structural change to create a different allele; the new allele resulting from such a change

**MZ**: monozygotic

**N**: haploid number of chromosomal DNA double-helices; in humans, 23

**neoplasia**: ability of cancerous cells to proliferate in defiance of normal controls

**NHC protein**: non-histone chromosomal protein

**NOR**: nucleolar organizer region

**NTD**: neural tube defect

**nucleoside**: compound of a purine or pyrimidine base linked to the sugar ribose or deoxyribose, e.g. adenosine, guanosine, cytidine, thymidine, uridine

**nucleotide**: compound of a purine or pyrimidine base linked to ribose or deoxyribose, plus phosphoric acid, e.g. d-adenosine triphosphate, d-ATP

**O**: blood group O

**obligate carrier**: individual who, logically, must be a carrier

**oligogenic**: resulting from the joint action of a small number of genes

**oligonucleotide**: artificially synthesized DNA molecule

**oncogene**: a modified proto-oncogene that contributes to a high rate of cell division, usually designated without a prefix, e.g. *myc*

**outbreeding**: breeding with an unrelated partner

**P**: degree of penetrance

**p**: chromosomal short arm; symbol for allele frequency

**p53**: mitosis suppressor protein product of the gene, *TP53*

**PCR**: polymerase chain reaction

**penetrance**: proportion of individuals of a specific genotype that shows the expected phenotype

**pharmacogenetics**: the aspect of genetics that deals with variation in response to drugs

**pharmacogenomics**: production of drugs by use of genetically engineered microorganisms

**phase**: of linkage, the state of association of alternative alleles at one locus with those at a genetically linked locus

**phenotype**: visible, tangible, or otherwise measurable properties of an organism resulting from the interaction of his or her genes with the environment

**PKU**: phenylketonuria

**pleiotropy**: phenomenon of a single gene being responsible for a number of distinct and often seemingly unrelated phenotypic traits

**point mutation**: substitution, insertion or deletion in DNA that involves only a small number of nucleotides

**Pol II**: RNA polymerase II

**polygenic**: resulting from the joint action of two or more genes

**polymorphism**: presence in a population of two or more alleles at one locus at frequencies each greater than 1%; one allele of a polymorphic system, or its corresponding phenotype

**premutation**: situation where there is expansion of triplet repeats beyond the normal range, but insufficient to cause disease

**preventive genetics**: application of genetic insight for avoidance of disease

**proband**: family member with specific phenotype who first came to the attention of the investigator or clinician

**proposita**: female proband

**propositus**: male proband

**proto-oncogene**: cellular oncogene; a normal allele that stimulates cell division, designated with the prefix 'c', e.g. c-myc

**pseudo-autosomal region**: similar region of the X and Y chromosomes where crossover occurs

**P–WS**: Prader–Willi syndrome

**q**: chromosomal long arm; symbol for allele frequency

**R-bands**: reverse bands, GC-rich parts of chromosomes that do not stain darkly with Giemsa stain, c.f. G-bands

**'rare'**: of genetic diseases, usually considered as occurring in less than 1/5000 births

**recessive**: an allele is said to be recessive to an alternative allele at the same locus when its expression is masked by that alternative in a heterozygote

**recurrence risk**: risk a couple will have another child with the same disorder

**repulsion**: 'trans' conformation

**restriction endonuclease**: enzyme that specifically cuts double-stranded DNA at a defined base sequence

**restriction fragment**: portion of double-stranded DNA released when DNA is cut with a restriction endonuclease

**reverse transcriptase**: viral enzyme that creates DNA copies from a RNA template

**RFLP**: restriction fragment length polymorphism

**RNA**: ribonucleic acid

**rRNA**: ribosomal RNA

**S**: Svedberg unit; DNA synthetic phase of the cell cycle.

**sarcoma**: malignant tumor of mesodermal tissue

**SCID**: severe combined immunodeficiency disease

**sense strand**: DNA strand complementary to the template strand and of sequence similar to that in the RNA transcribed

**sex chromosomes**: X and Y chromosomes

**sex limitation**: sex-related expression of an autosomal gene due to sex-related differences in anatomy or physiology

**sex linkage**: inheritance and expression of an allele in relation to sex, by virtue of the gene being carried on a sex chromosome

**silent mutation**: mutation that causes no change in the corresponding polypeptide

**sister chromatids**: two daughter strands of a duplicated chromosome joined by a common centromere

**snRNA**: small nuclear RNA

*SRY*: male sex determining gene

**SSCP**: single strand conformation polymorphism; study of DNA polymorphism by electrophoresis of DNA denatured into single strands

**snRNP**: small nuclear ribonucleo-protein; protein-RNA complex important in recognition of intron/exon boundaries, intron excision, or exon splicing, etc.

**somatic mutation**: mutation that occurs in a body cell

**START signal**: triplet codon AUG that signifies where translation of mRNA should start

**STC**: signal transduction cascade

**STOP signal**: chain terminator, or 'nonsense codon'; triplet codon that indicates where on the mRNA translation should stop: UAA, UAG, UGA

**susceptibility gene**: gene with an allele that confers predisposition to a disease

**synapsis**: side-by-side association of homologous chromosomes at meiosis

**syndrome**: set of phenotypic features that occur together as a characteristic of a disease

**T**: thymine; trisomy

**tandem repeats**: two or more copies of the same sequence of nucleotides arranged in direct succession in DNA

**TCA cycle**: tricarboxylic acid cycle

**telomere**: specialized end of a chromosome

**template strand**: anti-sense strand; the DNA strand along which RNA polymerase runs, producing an RNA molecule of complementary sequence

**test mating**: mating with a recessive homozygote which reveals the genotype of that individual

**threshold trait**: a character which shows discontinuous variation considered to be superimposed upon a continuously variable distribution of liabilities

*TP53*: the gene coding for protein p53

**trans conformation**: alleles of two linked genes are said to be in *trans* conformation when they are on opposite chromosomes at meiosis, c.f. *cis*

**transcript**: initially formed RNA polymerase product of the action of RNA

**translocation**: mutation that involves transfer of a piece of DNA to an abnormal site

**tRNA**: transfer RNA

**triplet repeat**: tandem repetition of a group of three bases in DNA

**tumour suppressor gene**: mitosis suppressor gene; a gene responsible for arresting mitosis at the G1 or G2 block

**U**: uracil

**UCL**: unilateral cleft lip

**viral oncogene**: oncogene derived from a viral insert, designated with the prefix 'v', e.g. v-myc

**VNTR**: variable number tandem repeat; usually applied to minisatellites

**zinc finger protein**: a protein of specialized structure stabilized by an atom of zinc with the property of binding to specific DNA sequences

# Appendix: Information resources

## Introductory general textbooks

Connor M, Ferguson-Smith M. *Essential Medical Genetics*, 5th edn. Oxford: Blackwell, 1997.

Cummings MR. *Human Heredity, Principles and Issues*, 5th edn. Pacific Grove, California: Brooks/Cole, 2000.

Gelehrter TD, Collins FS, Ginsburg D. *Principles of Medical Genetics*, 2nd edn. Baltimore: Williams and Wilkins, 1997.

Korf, BR. *Human Genetics. A Problem-Based Approach*, 2nd edn. Boston: Blackwell Science, 2000.

Mueller RF, Young ID. *Emery's Elements of Medical Genetics*, 11th edn. Edinburgh: Churchill Livingstone, 2001.

Nussbaum RL, McInnes RR, Willard HF. *Thompson and Thompson Genetics in Medicine*, 6th edn. Philadelphia: WB Saunders, 2001.

## Advanced general textbooks

Rimoin DL, Connor JM, Pyeritz RE, Korf BR. *Emery and Rimoin's Principles and Practice of Medical Genetics, Vols 1-3*, 4th edn. London: Churchill Livingstone, 2002.

Childs B, Beaudet AL, Valle D, Kinzler KW, Vogelstein B. *The Metabolic and Molecular Bases of Inherited Disease, Vols 1-4*, Eds: Scriver CR, Sly WS. New York: McGraw-Hill, 2000.

## Specialized textbooks

Emery AEH. *Methodology in Medical Genetics. An Introduction to Statistical Methods*, 2nd edn. Edinburgh: Churchill Livingstone, 1986.

Emery AEH, Malcolm S. *An Introduction to Recombinant DNA in Medicine*, 2nd edn. Wiley: Chichester, 1995.

Harper P. *Practical Genetic Counselling*, 5th edn. Oxford: Butterworth Heinemann, 1998.

Winter RM, Baraitser M. *Multiple Congenital Anomalies. A Diagnostic Compendium*. London: Chapman and Hall, 1991.

Evett IW, Weir BS. *Interpreting DNA Evidence. Statistical Genetics for Forensic Scientists*. Sunderland, Massachusetts: Sinauer, 1998.

## Internet databases

**Allele Frequency Database (ALFRED)**: http://alfred.med.yale.edu/alfred/index.asp

Makes available frequency data on single nucleotide polymorphisms (SNPs) in specific populations, linking these to the molecular genetics-human genome databases.

**Clinical Genetics Computer Resources**: http://www.kumc.edu/gec/prof/genecomp.html

A valuable entry point to all the major genetics databases, for professional use.

**Frequency of Inherited Disorders Database (FIDD)**: http://archive.uwcm.ac.uk/uwcm/mg/fidd/background.html

A compendium of published data on prevalence and incidence of diseases in human populations.

**GeneReviews**: http://genereviews.org

Database of laboratories that perform molecular diagnosis for specific disorders, plus an online genetics textbook with reviews and educational materials, including guidelines for diagnosis and management of genetic conditions.

**Genetic Alliance**: http://www.geneticalliance.org

Organization of support groups for genetic disorders, a good source of information for families.

**Human Mutation Database**: http://www.hgmd.org

A compendium of databases of mutations responsible for human genetic disorders.

**Infobiogen Database Catalogue (DBCAT)**: http://www.infobiogen.fr/services/dbcat/

Comprehensive public catalogue of biological databases.

**Online Mendelian Inheritance in Man (OMIM):** USA: http://www.ncbi.nlm.nih.gov/omim/; UK: http://www.hgmp.mrc.ac.uk/omim/

The standard and authoritative source of current knowledge of single gene disorders. Presents links to relevant literature, map locations and clinical summaries.

**PubMed**: http://www.ncbi.nlm.nih.gov/entrez/query.fcgi?db=PubMed

A service of the National Library of Medicine providing access to 11 million MEDLINE citations of standard publications on medical topics.

**The Family Village**: http://www.familyvillage.wisc.edu/

Source of information on medical disorders, targeted at the general public.

**The National Center for Biotechnology Information**: http://www.ncbi.nlm.nih.gov/

Provides links to many valuable genetic resources.

# Index